Table of Contents

T5-DHD-066

Table of Contents, *continued*

Illustrations by Margaret Warner and Eulala Conner
Page Layout by Christine Buysse, Cover Design by Mike Paustian

Introduction

How the *Let's Get Ready* Program Got Started

Though we were both therapists treating the same children in the same early intervention preschool, we didn't actually become acquainted until our therapy treatment days overlapped purely by chance. Before then, our therapy approaches and our individual goals were not coordinated or integrated.

When we finally began working on the same days, we recognized the relationship between our professional domains. We began to observe each other's treatment sessions and techniques. We noticed that the children we serviced benefited from a multidisciplinary approach. It was at this time that we realized that we could design a therapy "curriculum" that would access and integrate the knowledge in both speech and occupational therapy concurrently. The sum would be greater than its parts! Using a child-friendly puppet as a mascot, the Let's Get Ready *group was conceived.*

The current treatment delivery model in many early intervention classrooms consists of contracted therapists and staff therapists who usually function independently of each other. Therapy services are provided on different days and sometimes in different parts of the building. There is no collaboration time set aside for therapists to interact and coordinate therapy goals and objectives. Sometimes therapists who service children on different days do not even meet for months.

Our group, designed for preschool special needs classrooms with related therapies, initiates a new integrative therapeutic approach. The program emphasizes speech and occupational therapy goals with additional support from the physical therapist. In general, the speech-language pathologist (SLP) directs the oral motor activities and the occupational therapist (OT) runs the activities that are related to fine motor and postural control. The classroom teacher and any assistants are involved in the program by being in the room to assist the children during the activities.

Teachers have a monthly curriculum that generally follows the developmental continuum, so why can't therapists? The *Let's Get Ready* program provides a month-by-month guide for speech and occupational therapists that moves along the progression of the acquisition of oral motor and fine motor skills. The school year begins with basic motor foundational skills central to the achievement of both oral motor and fine motor development. As the months progress, the two disciplines diverge to emphasize the higher level specific skills necessary in each domain for success in functional language and fine motor activities.

Benefits

The purpose of the *Let's Get Ready* program is to provide an opportunity for maximizing the interrelationship of therapists and therapy goals in an easy-to-use organized monthly progression. There are numerous benefits to the program:

1. It is conducted in the classroom and includes all classroom staff. This aspect fits with the prevailing push for therapists to treat in "natural environments" and to involve the whole team. The key benefit is that teachers, assistants, and therapists learn to use and carry over therapy techniques of each specialty. The SLP, for example, can learn to watch how children use their wrists to turn over "beginning sound" cards, while the OT can listen for the final consonant as the children shout "POP" when popping bubbles. Additionally, without direct instruction, teachers, and assistants can pick up therapy strategies. The classroom staff can learn therapy techniques and ideas without confrontational corrections and comments from therapists, which leads to better personal relationships among all team members.

2. The curriculum follows the continuum of both speech and occupational therapy domains, from basic postural and trunk body movements to discrete fine and oral motor movements. The program can be visualized as a sturdy tree, with physical therapy at the base and roots. The trunk of the tree incorporates both speech and occupational therapy which are superimposed on a base of stable body and basic motor-planning skills. Fundamentals such as breath control and trunk elongation interrelate at the broad mid-trunk as a foundation for both speech and OT. Further up the tree, speech therapy and occupational therapy branch off, each leading to the higher level activities in their own domains. This allows the tree to truly "flower" with oral motor and fine motor competencies.

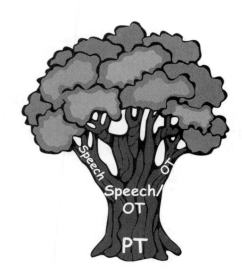

3. The program bridges that mysterious gap between a clinical service delivery model and an educational one. As a therapist using this curriculum, you will be able to work on those crucial foundational aspects of your discipline through targeted, clinically therapeutic activities. Yet the "destination point" of the program is clearly educationally relevant, functional competencies. Some of the specific tasks, such as pronouncing consonants and carrying a cafeteria tray, are common functional IEP goals. Other activities serve more as mileposts on the developmental continuum, but all are essential for skill acquisition and typical age functioning in speech and occupational therapy domains.

　　　　　　　　　　6　　　　　　　　　Copyright © 2004 LinguiSystems, Inc.

4. *Let's Get Ready* is a crowd pleaser! Parents love the team interaction and clinical therapeutic aspects of the program that go hand-in-hand with its functional outcomes for their children. Administrators appreciate its low cost and the way several treatments interface, causing less disruption to the regular school program. Teachers enjoy giving the command over to other professionals for a short time each week. And of course, the kids can never get enough of the Buzzy Bee puppet!

5. The program acts as a social connector. It fosters social interaction among the children as well as among the children, therapists, and classroom staff. It also provides a regular built-in routine for the children and staff that everyone anticipates and depends on.

6. The program uses highly motivational, fun activities and manipulatives to meet treatment goals. Most props in the program are household or low-cost items that are in your home or school setting.

7. The program gets the children ready to learn, but it is also ready for you, the therapist! The therapy curriculum details therapy themes month by month and activities week by week. After you accumulate a month's worth of activity supplies, you can walk in and lead an organized, therapeutically sound, interdisciplinary group with little planning. If the program is used for subsequent years, you can even further reduce planning time.

8. The program provides the speech and occupational therapy interventions listed on page 18, but there are also additional, less obvious communication and motor aspects that occur throughout each session. Group time provides on-going verbal and nonverbal communication learning opportunities for the children. And correct positioning and refining movement patterns are incorporated throughout each and every group activity. The program is truly not just multidisciplinary, but interdisciplinary at its core.

In summary, the *Let's Get Ready* program is a unique opportunity for children to have fun while strengthening their oral motor, fine motor, and sensory motor skills. It simultaneously benefits children, classroom staff, therapists, administrators, and parents.

What exactly is the *Let's Get Ready* program?

The *Let's Get Ready* program is a weekly therapeutic intervention implemented for approximately 15-25 minutes. The group follows a predictable routine each week. It starts with a greeting by our mascot, Buzzy Bee (a bee puppet). All puppets are appealing, but the bee puppet makes a noise (squeaker in its mouth) and has a moving part (wings). Therefore, it supplies maximum visual and auditory stimuli. The puppet is used intermittently during the group session to help refocus the children's attention and to transition between different activities.

7 Copyright © 2004 LinguiSystems, Inc.

Introduction, *continued*

The greeting is followed by a warm-up sensory motor activity that is combined with a language component to establish the therapeutic theme for the month. Next, the specific speech and occupational therapy activities are implemented. Even though each therapist has certain objectives, both therapists and the classroom staff assist in implementing each activity. The monthly themes follow a specific developmental progression, starting in the fall with more basic, whole body activities and ending in the spring with higher level, discrete tasks. According to the children's developmental levels and type of disabilities, the activities can be varied to meet their needs. The children participate in different activities for each week that coordinate with the overall monthly theme. The bee puppet is used throughout the activities in a variety of ways. (Specific ideas are listed in the next question.)

To enhance language, you can ask basic *who, what, where, when, why,* and *how* questions. Language prompts are included for those activities we felt needed to focus on a specific type of question or concept. Other language prompts could focus on size, quantity, colors, and concepts (e.g., *over, under, first, last*).

Your own creativity and experience can add to the success of the *Let's Get Ready* program. Feel free to supplement each month's activities with your own ideas related to the monthly developmental themes. You may want to choose manipulative items that coordinate with a specific classroom project or lesson. You may already have some interesting toys or pieces of equipment that can be adapted. Extra activities for each month are provided in the book. These extra activities can reinforce the month's goals and lengthen the sessions if your students can tolerate a longer group. Activity calendars for the months of July and August are also provided to reinforce therapy skills learned during the year.

How is the bee puppet used in this program?

The bee puppet can be used many ways during a session. You will want to keep the puppet within arm's reach so you can access it quickly.

- Use the puppet to initiate the therapy session.

  > Teacher to group of children: "Today is Monday. Who is the special friend that visits us on Mondays?"
  >
  > Children: "Buzzy Bee! It's the day Buzzy Bee comes!"
  >
  > Teacher: "Yes, today is the day that Buzzy Bee comes to play with you. Let's all listen to hear if he is ready to come out and play."

Then the SLP, who has the puppet hidden behind her back, makes him squeak. This engages the auditory attention of the children and prepares them for the start of the group. Buzzy Bee appears (visual stimulus) and the session begins (start with the Greeting).

　　　　　　Copyright © 2004 LinguiSystems, Inc.

- Squeak the bee to refocus the children's attention during an activity or game. You can also squeak the bee to transition between targeted tasks.

- Use the bee as a prompt to initiate a child's turn or to provide verbal and/or nonverbal cues.

- Use the bee's mouth as a target location for placing therapy manipulatives used in an activity (e.g., have the children give the bee a picture card rather than putting it in a box).

A few words from the physical therapist

I feel that my regular participation in the Let's Get Ready *group is a valuable use of my treatment time. I focus on the children on my caseload in the classroom, but my input on their behalf tacitly affects all of the kids by example. None of the activities can be successful without adequate postural support and proper body alignment. I advise and help in these areas, as well as the motor planning, balance, and strength requirements for each game. For me, seeing the relationship between PT goals and oral motor/fine motor skill acquisition has been revealing. For example, one child who was limited in trunk elongation was unable to produce adequate breath for speech. Another advantage of the* Let's Get Ready *program is that I can demonstrate positioning strategies to the classroom staff without actually having to point out what others are doing wrong. This leads to better carryover of my treatment goals in the classroom.*

Who is the *Let's Get Ready* program designed to help?

This program is designed for children enrolled in non-categorical, early intervention classes. These classes typically have 10-12 children, a teacher, and two assistants. The children have various levels of developmental delay. The program can also be used in a variety of other settings. It can be adapted to fit the needs of children enrolled in autistic/pervasive developmental disorder classes. This program can be structured to accommodate older children with moderate and severe levels of developmental delay. The program can also work as a support program for a learning support primary class in a typical school setting if a number of the children receive related services.

Finally, this program can be adapted for children who are physically handicapped or in wheelchairs by making individual adjustments based on their physical limitations. Children in wheelchairs can do many of the postural activities using only their upper bodies. Objects may need to be positioned on a tray or table rather than on the floor.

How much will it cost to do the *Let's Get Ready* program?

Not much! Each month a variety of props are needed. These include items you may already have or can easily purchase (e.g., food, bubbles, ping-pong balls, plates). The items can be used year after year, with the exception of food and plastic utensils. Once you have your supplies, you're ready to run the program with no significant further expenses.

Program Assessment

The *Let's Get Ready* program's usefulness can be maximized if you take a few minutes to review each session at its conclusion. Each week, you should assess the effectiveness of each activity and consider how the activity can be modified to better meet the needs of your specific population. This is particularly important for the warm-up activities, which are repeated throughout the month. You can refer to your completed *Data Tracking Sheets* (page 140) to determine if any specific accommodations need to be made to meet the needs of individual students. In addition, you should ask for and take into account feedback from the classroom staff. During this review time, also take a few minutes to look ahead at the activities listed for the next week. Make sure the supplies are available. Decide if the activities are likely to be successful with your group, or whether you need to increase or decrease the level of challenge. These simple strategies will help maintain a high level of quality and efficacy in your sessions.

How will the *Let's Get Ready* program help you formulate IEP goals?

The developmental progression of speech and OT themes and their related rationales in the *Let's Get Ready* program can be readily translated into IEP goals for the children on your caseload. To accomplish this, you will need to carefully observe each child you treat during the program's activities. The *Data Tracking Sheet* (page 140) will assist you in identifying specific problem areas for each child. You can use this data sheet and your own testing and/or clinical observations to assess each child's individual needs.

To use a *Let's Get Ready* theme/rationale as the basis for an IEP goal, you will need to expand upon that theme/rationale to make it specific and measurable for an individual child. A measurable annual goal should answer the following questions:

- Who will achieve the goal?
- What skill or behavior will be achieved?
- How will the goal be achieved? (In what manner or at what level?)
- Where will the skill occur?

Depending on the IEP format in your setting, you may then need to design benchmark objectives that relate to your annual goal. These are measurable, discrete tasks that will enable you to determine if the annual goal has been met. Example goals for speech and OT are on the next page.

Copyright © 2004 LinguiSystems, Inc.

Here are some examples of generic and individualized goals for speech and OT:

Speech	OT
Theme: tongue elevation	**Theme:** bilateral motor skills and midline crossing
Rationale Tongue elevation activities will help in strengthening the tip of the tongue. Tongue elevation is essential for the production of /t, d, n, s, l, z/ and /ch/ in words, phrases, sentences, and conversational speech.	**Rationale** To develop a skillful dominant hand, children must be able to cross the midline of the body in activities. A well-established dominant hand is necessary to achieve fine motor control. The non-dominant hand is also important to stabilize objects as the dominant hand performs an activity. Therefore, the children must acquire bilateral integration as well as midline crossing.
Generic Goals (Name of child) will achieve tongue elevation. (Name of child) will strengthen oral musculature. (Name of child) will produce sounds that require tongue elevation.	**Generic Goals** (Name of child) will demonstrate progress in bilateral motor skills. (Name of child) will exhibit midline crossing during activities.
Individualized Goals (Add *what, how,* and *where* to your goals.) Kelci will demonstrate progress in tongue elevation exercises during classroom activities with a member of the team and/or peer by imitating movements of the tongue with verbal and visual prompts with 80% accuracy. Kelci will produce the target phonemes /t/ and /d/ in the initial position of monosyllabic syllables and words after a model by imitating tongue elevation during individualized and group therapy sessions with 80% accuracy.	**Individualized Goals** (Add *what, how,* and *where* to your goals.) Tasha will demonstrate progress in bilateral motor skills in the classroom art activities by using standard child-sized scissors to cut across a six-inch paper square, maintaining her nondominant hand on the paper to stabilize it with one or fewer verbal prompts. Tasha will exhibit midline crossing in prewriting activities in the classroom by independently drawing a horizontal line across a paper with a supinated grasp on a crayon using only her dominant hand when given a demonstration.

Copyright © 2004 LinguiSystems, Inc.

Introduction, *continued*

Think of how your benchmark objectives can lead progressively up to your annual goal. Use this program to help you both *assess* and *work on* problem areas that you observe in the children. The activities in this program will clearly highlight the children who have trouble with a specific task. The activities will also give you an opportunity to practice the foundational skills necessary to achieve each activity in a therapeutic, fun format. You can use therapy time with a child later in the day to continue to individually practice skills that were difficult for him during the group session. Since the entire classroom team is part of the program, other staff members can also continue to practice during any available or appropriate class time.

To **decrease** the level of expectation for a child's annual goals, change the following variables:

- Decrease the number of expected successful trials (e.g., move from 90% accuracy to 60% accuracy).

- Use a less-demanding tool (e.g., use spring or loop scissors instead of regular scissors for an OT cutting goal).

- Add more therapist prompts (e.g., increase the number of verbal prompts; use a variety of prompts such as verbal, tactile, or visual).

- Add more physical support (e.g., provide adapted seating with more postural support, attach a tray onto a wheelchair for manipulatives such as pictures or objects).

- Change the manipulatives:

    ✓ move from abstract to concrete examples
    ✓ use objects instead of pictures
    ✓ pair objects with picture symbols
    ✓ use a slant board (a board with a 90-degree angle) for displaying flash cards or to stabilize paper
    ✓ use materials that provide less physical resistance (e.g., softer clay)
    ✓ use fine motor manipulatives that are larger in size and therefore, easier to handle

To **increase** the level of expectation for a child's annual goal, change the following variables:

- Increase the number of expected successful trials (e.g., move from 70% to 80% accuracy or from 80% to 90% accuracy).

- Increase the complexity of the old behavior by adding a challenge:

    ✓ produce the target sound in words from syllables
    ✓ produce the target sound in phrases from words

✓ produce the target sound in sentences from phrases
✓ produce the target sound in spontaneous speech from modeled speech
✓ increase the number of steps in a fine motor task
✓ increase the speed requirement for fine motor activities

- Develop a new behavior to target (e.g., the child mastered the production of /t/. Start remediation on the production of /d/.).

- Decrease prompts from the therapist.

- Decrease the number of expected errors over a specified time period (e.g., with two or fewer errors over a 10-minute period).

- Change the manipulatives (e.g., use more complex or resistive materials).

- Work on the same goal for a longer period of time.

- Include new partners (e.g., expand who the child needs to practice with, such as teachers, therapists, peers, cafeteria workers, bus drivers, parents, siblings).

A few words from the authors

As therapists, the Let's Get Ready *program has truly improved our service delivery. We have a ready-made, organized progression of therapeutic activities to use in the group we lead each week. This program highlights specific oral motor and fine motor difficulties of individual children, helping us target treatment goals carefully and appropriately. And, by using this program, we have learned to add components of one another's domains to our independent therapy treatments (e.g., Michelle is more comfortable positioning picture cards at the table to require forearm supination and pronation, while Fern is able to choose manipulative items with more appropriate speech sound requirements for specific children). This kind of knowledge enables us to treat the whole child more effectively.*

We hope you have fun with the activities in the *Let's Get Ready* program. Our children, classroom staff, and therapists (e.g., speech, occupational, physical) look forward to the weekly sessions. And parents and administrators who come to observe, love the program, which is a marriage between both the clinical and educational models of service delivery that actually works in a classroom setting!

Fern and Michelle

13 Copyright © 2004 LinguiSystems, Inc.

Materials List

Here is a list of materials needed for the entire *Let's Get Ready* program. Materials for each month are also listed on the first page of each month throughout the book. You will have many of these items in your classroom already. For consumable items such as gift wrap tubes or empty spice containers, send notes home with your children. Parents are a great resource!

Remember to review all children's files for allergies to food products and/or dietary restrictions before doing any activities in this program.

October			
Each week you will need Buzzy Bee and a 10"-12" playground ball.			
Week One	**Week Two**	**Week Three**	**Week Four**
bottle of bubbles chair box of tissues 9 Ping-Pong balls	Styrofoam plates scissors cotton balls straws	pencil 2 bottles of bubbles	broom or broom handle scooter board hula hoop pinwheel white tissue paper Ping-Pong ball piece of string marker

November			
Each week you will need Buzzy Bee, a small tray with handles, and objects/pictures for the tray.			
Week One	**Week Two**	**Week Three**	**Week Four**
2 cube chairs chewy treats (e.g., gummy candy, fruit snacks)	4 (or more) coffee cans with plastic lids items for the coffee cans (e.g., pennies, marshmallows, blocks, jelly beans) mirror Goldfish crackers plastic gloves (non-latex)	play parachute chewy treats (e.g., gummy candy, fruit snacks, jelly beans)	18"-22" therapy ball child-sized backpack several cans of food portable clinic stairs or access to stairs licorice sticks (2 different colors/flavors) plastic gloves (non-latex)

January			
Each week you will need Buzzy Bee.			
Week One	**Week Two**	**Week Three**	**Week Four**
3 bathroom-sized paper cups 3 stickers tongue depressors or straws 2½" x ½" pretzel dipping sticks	pairs of animal flash cards empty toilet paper rolls uncooked macaroni clear packing tape stickers straws Froot Loops party blowers small zippered bags permanent marker	hand lotion animal stickers hand puppets (at least 4) Cheerios coffee stirrers	variety of small wind-up toys several empty plastic spice containers M&Ms lip balm cotton swabs tongue depressors pennies tape

February			
Each week you will need Buzzy Bee.			
Week One	**Week Two**	**Week Three**	**Week Four**
3 coffee cans with plastic lids long-handled spoons or drumsticks beanbags bathroom-sized paper cups plastic spoons thawed Cool Whip	stickers 6 colorful beanbags therapy barrel sandwich cookies (e.g., Oreos)	Stryrofoam plates from October yardstick construction paper or thematic pictures scissors masking tape colorful seals (lick-and-stick) jar of peanut butter Ritz crackers plastic knife paper plate	2 child-sized chairs 2 empty gift wrap tubes 1 beanbag animal crackers 2 squeeze tubes of different flavored icing paper plate or small plastic container

Materials List, *continued*

March			
Each week you will need Buzzy Bee and two different-colored sponges cut in half.			
Week One	**Week Two**	**Week Three**	**Week Four**
2 chairs 2 small spray bottles paper towels paper of various types and textures basket (for target) picture of a snowman easel or masking tape beach ball permanent marker	carpet squares 2 clear plastic containers 2 regular-sized sponges paper towels small table 2 sheets of construction paper flash cards (or objects) that begin with /p/* flash cards (or objects) that begin with /b/* box	2 small suitcases with rigid handles 2 child-sized chairs objects of various weights small, smooth toys (e.g., balls, rubber animals, plastic beads) 2 sheets of construction paper flash cards (or objects) that begin with /t/* flash cards (or objects) that begin with /d/* play toolbox	large, soft rope blanket oranges knife strainer transparent pitcher 2 hand juicers small paper cups 2 sheets of construction paper flash cards (or objects) that begin with /m/* flash cards (or objects) that begin with /n/* play mailbox mirror

April			
Each week you will need Buzzy Bee, two washable markers, and smiley face stickers.			
Week One	**Week Two**	**Week Three**	**Week Four**
farm animal figures uncooked macaroni toy frying pan or pot wooden dowel (26" long) string magnet Mouth Position cards ** large paper clips	2 manila folders brown marker or crayon scissors 2 sheets of construction paper flash cards (or objects) that begin with /k/* flash cards (or objects) that begin with /g/* plastic bowling pins and balls tongue depressors mirror	teddy bear spring-type clothespins stickers of items beginning with initial sounds previously targeted shoebox classroom theme-related picture to color ink pad(s) tray or table construction paper scissors flash cards (or objects) that begin with /s/* Twister game beanbag	foil chewy treats clay, play dough, or Theraputty pennies child's purse with clasp or large change purse with clasp fishing pole (from Week One) 2 sheets of construction paper Sea Creatures*** flash cards that begin with /f/* flash cards that begin with /v/* large paper clips mirror

*See pages 143-154.   **See pages 168-172.   ***See pages 163-167.

May			
Each week you will need Buzzy Bee.			
Week One	**Week Two**	**Week Three**	**Week Four**
Froot Loops 2 small plastic bowls pipe cleaners masking tape small paper plates pencil plastic tray Cool Whip (thawed) wet paper towels small table plastic eggs basket (to hold the eggs) VC nonsense syllables*	2 baby dolls cotton balls stretchy men figures pennies dimes container (to hold the dimes) construction paper flash cards (or objects) that end with /p/** flash cards (or objects) that end with /b/** flash cards (or objects) that end with /m/**	plastic tray shaving cream wet paper towels several finger puppets construction paper 16 16-ounce plastic cups masking tape 3 Ping-Pong balls flash cards (or objects) that end with /k/** flash cards (or objects) that end with /g/** 2 plastic containers (for the flash cards) marker	bubble wrap plastic container with lid scissors permanent marker pennies treats (e.g., gummy candy, M&Ms) flash cards (or objects) that end with /s/** flash cards (or objects) that end with /t/** flash cards (or objects) that end with /d/**
June			
Week One			
Buzzy Bee vanilla and chocolate ice cream 2 ice-cream scoops plastic or Styrofoam bowls fudge and caramel syrup M&Ms chocolate and rainbow sprinkles in plastic shaker containers plastic spoons 2 small trays with handles napkins			

*See page 133.

**See pages 155-162.

Monthly Speech and OT Coordinated Themes

	Speech	OT
September	Getting Ready	Getting Ready
October	Breath Support	Trunk Elongation
November	Jaw Stabilization	Postural Control
December	Review	Review
January	Lip Closure	Wrist Control
February	Tongue Elevation	Bilateral Motor Skills Midline Crossing
March	Sound Recognition, Discrimination, and Pronunciation of Early-Developing Initial Sounds	Grasp
April	Sound Recognition, Discrimination, and Pronunciation of Later-Developing Initial Sounds	Finger Isolation Pincer Grasp
May	Sound Recognition, Discrimination, and Pronunciation of Previously Targeted Sounds in the Final Position	Separation of the Two Sides of the Hand In-hand Manipulation Skills
June	Celebration of Skills	Celebration of Skills
July	Activities for Skill Reinforcement	Activities for Skill Reinforcement
August	Activities for Skill Reinforcement	Activities for Skill Reinforcement

SEPTEMBER

Theme: Getting Ready

September in the *Let's Get Ready* program is designated for you to get to know the children and for the children to become accustomed to the classroom routine. For this reason, the actual *Let's Get Ready* curriculum is designed to begin in October rather than September. However, there are a number of factors to be examined and a variety of materials to assemble in September in order to properly prepare yourself, the children, and the classroom staff before the start of the program.

First, consider that at this initial early point in the school year, many children are not yet able to sit in a group and follow directions. For some students, this may be their first school experience. They might have difficulty separating from parents or participating in activities alongside their peers. For others, the physical environment or adults in the classroom may be new. Even different school transportation methods could be confusing to some children, such as riding on a school bus for the first time or being restrained in a different car seat by an unfamiliar bus driver.

It is important to have a feel for the individual needs of the children and the level of functioning in the classroom before initiating the *Let's Get Ready* curriculum. You will need to make a professional assessment of the degree of challenge necessary for the majority of students. Most of the activities can be graded up or down to increase or decrease the level of difficulty. You will also need to be familiar with the program so you can arrange an appropriate adult/child ratio in the group. Other things to consider include:

- Can the class participate in one large group, or would the program work better with the group split in half? If the class is split into two groups, you might want one group to have a higher level of challenge.

- How close together can the chairs be arranged so the children relate to each other as a group but personal boundaries are preserved?

- Are there any children who should not be seated next to each other during the group activities?

- Do any of the children require one-on-one assistance from a member of the classroom team?

To keep individual data on children during the program, you may want to make copies of the *Data Tracking Sheet* on page 140. This sheet can be prepared before the sessions so data collection is less cumbersome and disruptive. Consult with the classroom staff to see if they are willing to assist with data collection.

Copyright © 2004 LinguiSystems, Inc.

You also need to be familiar with the individual IEP goals in speech and occupational therapy for each child. September is a crucial month for matching each child to her particular goals, noting her strengths and needs. That way, the sessions can truly target the individual child. For example, a certain child may need extra physical prompts to position herself in a high kneel posture or to use both hands in an activity. Another student might need extra time to imitate vocal sounds and sequences or to respond to questions or commands.

September is also the month to acquire the supplies you'll need for the program. We suggest that you prepare at least half of the year's materials in advance, making a list of items you want to begin saving at home, such as plastic spice containers. Determine who is responsible for gathering specific items needed for the program. Make sure all materials gathered for the implementation of the program are placed in a plastic tote and kept in the classroom. Keep in mind that the process of accumulating your materials is only something you need to go through the first year. In subsequent years of using the program, you will merely have to make a quick review of items and an occasional food purchase to use the curriculum.

The physical setting should be analyzed, using guidance from the physical therapist if possible.

- Are there special seating or sensory requirements for any of the children? Some students may need a more supportive seating design if low tone issues are present. Others may benefit from sensory modifications, such as a weighted vest or an air-filled chair cushion to provide subtle movement when seated.

- How can the visibility of other materials, toys, or noise levels be minimized to create the most distraction-free environment possible in a school setting?

- If the classroom environment is inappropriate, are there other locations in the school building that would be more conducive for the implementation of the program? You may want to consider leading the activities in a hallway or vacant room if the classroom is too distracting. The wall in a hallway can be used for children to lean their backs against for extra postural support.

> **Before beginning this program, it is extremely important to learn of any dietary restrictions or food allergies, specifically dairy, chocolate, and peanuts (peanut butter), that the children have. A review of the children's files will indicate if any child is on a special or limited diet, possesses any swallowing issues, or is prone to aspiration on small food items. A careful review of the children's medically-related school information is <u>essential</u> since food items are used in this program.**

In September, you will be busy getting to know your caseload, gathering your supplies, getting familiar with the program, and basically "getting ready" to begin the *Let's Get Ready* curriculum. Use this time to your best advantage and "Let's Get Ready" for success!

OCTOBER

Themes: Breath Support

Trunk Elongation

Rationale

Speech: Trunk elongation is the basis for breath support, which is necessary for phonation.

OT: The ability to elongate the trunk is basic to upper extremity movement and subsequent control of the upper extremities.

Helpful Hints:

 Keep Buzzy Bee within arm's reach so you can quickly access it during the activities as needed.

 If behavior or attention is a problem, you may want to divide the children into two separate groups (or two lines, depending on the activity) to achieve more control of the group.

Materials:
Buzzy Bee
10"-12" playground ball
bottle of bubbles
chair (for adult to stand on while blowing bubbles)
box of tissues
nine Ping-Pong balls

Greeting:
Have Buzzy Bee greet each child individually by saying, "Hi, (child's name)." Encourage each child to respond appropriately to the puppet with verbal or nonverbal language.

> *Therapist:* "It's time to say hello to Buzzy Bee! Hi, Evan!"
> *Verbal Child:* "Hi, Buzzy!"

> *Therapist:* "It's time to say hello to Buzzy Bee! Hi, Jamal!"
> *Nonverbal Child:* Child must initiate eye contact and wave or smile.

Warm-Up Activity:
Call the children one at a time by name to form a line, either sitting or standing. When the children are ready, show the children how to pass the ball to the person behind you by lifting your arms up over your head with the ball in your hands.

Have the children lift their arms up over their heads. Stand in the front of the line and pass a lightweight playground ball over your head to the first child in the line. Have the child pass the ball over his head to the next child, who passes the ball over his head to the next child and so on, down the line. Support each child in fully extending his trunk while maintaining a stable body position. Encourage the children to keep their arms up as long as they can, taking individual motor abilities into consideration. In addition, provide verbal language prompts to enhance the activity.

Language prompts:
- Who is in front of you?
- Who is behind you?
- Where is the ball going? *(over my head)*
- Where are your arms? *(up high, up in the air)*
- What color is the ball?

When the ball reaches the last child, have him pass it to the other therapist who then leads the group in a final cheer of "1, 2, 3, Hurray!" Have the children elongate their trunks again as they raise their arms for the cheer.

Copyright © 2004 LinguiSystems, Inc.

Repeat the activity two or three times, depending on how well the children are paying attention.

Variations
1. Change the size, texture, and/or weight of the ball.
2. Change the children's body positions (e.g., sitting, standing, kneeling).

Activity 1: Bubbles

Have the children sit on the floor. Stand on a chair and introduce the activity as a "bubble race." Explain that you will blow some bubbles and the children have to watch the bubbles to see which one reaches the floor first. Blow some bubbles into the air. The children must use neck extension to visually track the bubbles to see which one reaches the floor first.

Then have a few children come to the front of the group. Instruct them to reach above their heads to pop the bubbles by clapping. Have the children who are still seated visually track the bubbles while waiting for their turns. Depending on the number of children, it may be helpful to have two adults blowing bubbles.

Language prompts:
*   Where are the bubbles? *(in the bottle)*
*   Should the bubbles stay in the bottle?
*   What should I do? *(open bubbles, take lid off)*
*   Who is blowing the bubbles?
*   Where is (name of therapist) standing? *(on the chair)*
*   (Have your eyes closed.) Can I see the bubbles? *(no)*
    What should I do? *(open your eyes)*
*   Are (name of child)'s eyes open?
*   Are the bubbles sticky?

Activity 2: Blowing

Transition the children to tables and chairs. When the children are ready, show them how to take a deep breath and blow. Have the children practice blowing. Then hold a tissue with two hands in front of your face and make it move by blowing. Have each child reach for a tissue from a box held above his head to further facilitate trunk extension. Then have the child practice blowing the tissue. After a few minutes, collect the tissues and throw them away.

Next, get one Ping-Pong ball. Kneel on the floor in front of a table and demonstrate how to blow the ball across the table to a child. Put one ball on each table for the children to blow across the table. Once the children have practiced blowing one ball, introduce a second and third ball to the table.

Week One, *continued*

Language prompts:
- What are you holding? *(a tissue)*
- Is the tissue hard or soft?
- What color is the tissue?
- Did your tissue move?
- What color is the ball?
- Is the ball heavy or light?
- Did you blow the ball?
- Who did you blow the ball to?
- Is the ball big or little?

Variation: Move the tissue further from the child's lips. This will force the child to inhale and take a deeper breath and thus blow for a longer period of time.

Wrap-Up: Reintroduce the bee puppet to end the group, say good-bye to the children, and direct them to the next classroom activity.

> Therapist: *"We're all finished! Let's say good-bye to Buzzy. Now it's time for (name of next classroom activity)."*

The classroom teacher then gives the children instructions about the next activity.

Copyright © 2004 LinguiSystems, Inc.

Week Two

Materials: Buzzy Bee
10"-12" playground ball
Styrofoam plates with the centers cut out
cotton balls
straws

Greeting: Have Buzzy Bee greet each child individually by saying, "Hi, (child's name)." Encourage each child to respond appropriately to the puppet with verbal or nonverbal language.

> *Therapist:*   *"It's time to say hello to Buzzy Bee! Hi, Evan!"*
> *Verbal Child:*   *"Hi, Buzzy!"*

> *Therapist:*   *"It's time to say hello to Buzzy Bee! Hi, Jamal!"*
> *Nonverbal Child:*   *Child must initiate eye contact and wave or smile.*

Warm-Up Activity: Call the children one at a time by name to form a line, either sitting or standing. When the children are ready, show the children how to pass the ball to the person behind you by lifting your arms up over your head with the ball in your hands.

Have the children lift their arms up over their heads. Stand in the front of the line and pass a lightweight playground ball over your head to the first child in the line. Have the child pass the ball over his head to the next child, who passes the ball over his head to the next child and so on, down the line. Support each child in fully extending his trunk while maintaining a stable body position. Encourage the children to keep their arms up as long as they can, taking individual motor abilities into consideration. In addition, provide verbal language prompts to enhance the activity.

Language prompts:
- Who is in front of you?
- Who is behind you?
- Where is the ball going? *(over my head)*
- Where are your arms? *(up high, up in the air)*
- What color is the ball?

When the ball reaches the last child, have him pass it to the other therapist who then leads the group in a final cheer of "1, 2, 3, Hurray!" Have the children elongate their trunks again as they raise their arms for the cheer.

Repeat the activity two or three times, depending on how well the children are paying attention.

Variations
1. Change the size, texture, and/or weight of the ball.
2. Change the children's body positions (e.g., sitting, standing, kneeling).

Activity 1: I Am a Tree

Have the children stand up with enough space between them to fully extend their arms. Explain that each child will pretend to be a tree, using his arms as tall branches. Encourage the children to practice extending their arms up in the air. Place "leaves" (plates with centers cut out) on each child's arms, making sure that children sustain upper body and arm extension.

Have the children practice waving their "branches" (arms) and blowing like the wind, thus combining breath support simultaneously with trunk elongation. After a few minutes, have the children shake their "leaves" to the ground.

Next kneel on the ground with your arms fully extended up and pretend to be a "tree." Have each child take a turn to reach for two leaves held by the other therapist. Then have the child reach to place the leaves on your "tree."

Language prompts:
- Where are your arms? *(up in the air, up high, next to my body, down)*
- Where are the leaves (plates)? *(on my arms, on my branches)*
- Who is wearing the leaves?
- Where are the leaves now? *(on the ground)*
- How many leaves do you have?
- What color are your leaves?

Variation: Have each child kneel with his body at a 90-degree angle (high kneel) and "walk" to get the leaves/place the leaves on the tree.

Activity 2: Blowing

Transition the children to tables and chairs. When they are ready, show them how to take a deep breath and blow. Have the children practice. Then demonstrate how to blow a cotton ball across the table. Give each child a cotton ball to blow to another child.

Next demonstrate how to blow through a straw and feel the air coming through on the other side. Give each child a straw so he can practice. Then model how to blow through the straw to move the cotton ball. Have the children blow the cotton balls through their straws to the other children.

Language prompts:
- Where is the cotton ball? *(on the table, in my hand)*
- What color is the cotton ball?
- Is the cotton ball hard or soft?
- Can you squeeze the cotton ball?
- What do you need now? *(a straw)*
- Did you feel the air?
- What color is your straw?

Variations
1. Vary the length of the straw. A shorter straw requires the child to use a quick burst of air to move the cotton ball. A longer straw requires a longer continuous flow of air.
2. Have the children kneel at the table instead of sitting.

Wrap-Up: Reintroduce the bee puppet to end the group, say good-bye to the children, and direct them to the next classroom activity.

Therapist: *"We're all finished! Let's say good-bye to Buzzy. Now it's time for (name of next classroom activity)."*

The classroom teacher then gives the children instructions about the next activity.

Copyright © 2004 LinguiSystems, Inc.

Week Three

Materials: Buzzy Bee
10"-12" playground ball
pencil
two bottles of bubbles

Greeting: Have Buzzy Bee greet each child individually by saying, "Hi, (child's name)." Encourage each child to respond appropriately to the puppet with verbal or nonverbal language.

> *Therapist:*   *"It's time to say hello to Buzzy Bee! Hi, Evan!"*
> *Verbal Child:*   *"Hi, Buzzy!"*
>
> *Therapist:*   *"It's time to say hello to Buzzy Bee! Hi, Jamal!"*
> *Nonverbal Child:*   *Child must initiate eye contact and wave or smile.*

Warm-Up Activity: Call the children one at a time by name to form a line, either sitting or standing. When the children are ready, show the children how to pass the ball to the person behind you by lifting your arms up over your head with the ball in your hands.

Have the children lift their arms up over their heads. Stand in the front of the line and pass a lightweight playground ball over your head to the first child in the line. Have the child pass the ball over his head to the next child, who passes the ball over his head to the next child and so on, down the line. Support each child in fully extending his trunk while maintaining a stable body position. Encourage the children to keep their arms up as long as they can, taking individual motor abilities into consideration. In addition, provide verbal language prompts to enhance the activity.

Language prompts:
- Who is in front of you?
- Who is behind you?
- Where is the ball going? *(over my head)*
- Where are your arms? *(up high, up in the air)*
- What color is the ball?

When the ball reaches the last child, have him pass it to the other therapist who then leads the group in a final cheer of "1, 2, 3, Hurray!" Have the children elongate their trunks again as they raise their arms for the cheer.

Repeat the activity two or three times, depending on how well the children are paying attention.

Copyright © 2004 LinguiSystems, Inc.

Variations
1. Change the size, texture, and/or weight of the ball.
2. Change the children's body positions (e.g., sitting, standing, kneeling).

Activity 1: London Bridge

Have several pairs of children stand to form "bridges" with their arms extended overhead while holding hands with a partner. Have the other children form a line and pass under the "bridges" while the group sings the "London Bridge" song.

Language prompts:
- Where did you go? *(under the bridge)*
- Did you walk or crawl?

Variation: Have the children who form the "bridges" use a high kneel position on the floor. The other children can crawl through the bridges.

Activity 2: Log Roll

Explain that the children will "roll like pencils" across a carpeted section of the floor or on a therapy mat. Show how a real pencil rolls on a table. Then model a well-aligned body (log) roll with good trunk elongation and arm extension. Have each child come up to the front of the group and execute a log roll across the room. Encourage the children to keep their arms fully extended. The children may need a physical prompt on the hip and/or shoulder to initiate rolling. Provide verbal language prompts as needed. Reinforce the imagery of the pencil by explaining how the children's bodies are like pencils as they roll.

Language prompts:
- Who is rolling?
- Does (name of child) look like a pencil?
- Who rolled first? Last?

Activity 3: Cheek Popping

Take a deep breath, hold it, and fill your cheeks with air. Then describe what you did, including how your cheeks filled out like a balloon. Have the children practice filling their cheeks with air. Then demonstrate how to "pop" your cheeks with your index fingers. Have the children imitate several times.

Language prompts:
- Touch your cheeks.
- Did you pop your cheeks?
- Where did the air go?
- How did you pop your cheeks?

Activity 4: Blowing Bubbles

Bring out two bottles of soap bubbles. Demonstrate how to blow bubbles by taking a deep breath and releasing the air to blow the bubble off of the wand. Have two children blow bubbles at the same time while the other children encourage them to blow the bubbles.

Language prompts:
- What am I holding? *(bubbles)*
- What should I do? *(open them, take the lid off, blow)*
- Where is the bubble wand? *(in the bottle, inside)*
- Tell me what to do. *(take out the wand, blow)*
- (name of child), do you want to blow?

Variation: Move the wand further from the child's lips.

Wrap-Up: Reintroduce the bee puppet to end the group, say good-bye to the children, and direct them to the next classroom activity.

> Therapist: *"We're all finished! Let's say good-bye to Buzzy. Now it's time for (name of next classroom activity)."*

The classroom teacher then gives the children instructions about the next activity.

Materials: Buzzy Bee
10"-12" playground ball
broom or broom handle
scooter board
hula hoop
pinwheel
ghost (white tissue paper, Ping-Pong ball, piece of string or yarn, marker)

> (Note: The ghost is for the fourth activity. To make the ghost, put the Ping-Pong ball under a piece of tissue paper. Tie a piece of string under the ball to create the head. Make sure the string is long enough to suspend and swing the ghost. Draw a ghost face on the paper.)

Greeting: Have Buzzy Bee greet each child individually by saying, "Hi, (child's name)." Encourage each child to respond appropriately to the puppet with verbal or nonverbal language.

> *Therapist:* "It's time to say hello to Buzzy Bee! Hi, Evan!"
> *Verbal Child:* "Hi, Buzzy!"
>
> *Therapist:* "It's time to say hello to Buzzy Bee! Hi, Jamal!"
> *Nonverbal Child:* Child must initiate eye contact and wave or smile.

Warm-Up Activity: Call the children one at a time by name to form a line, either sitting or standing. When the children are ready, show the children how to pass the ball to the person behind you by lifting your arms up over your head with the ball in your hands.

Have the children lift their arms up over their heads. Stand in the front of the line and pass a lightweight playground ball over your head to the first child in the line. Have the child pass the ball over his head to the next child, who passes the ball over his head to the next child and so on, down the line. Support each child in fully extending his trunk while maintaining a stable body position. Encourage the children to keep their arms up as long as they can, taking individual motor abilities into consideration. In addition, provide verbal language prompts to enhance the activity.

Language prompts:
- Who is in front of you?
- Who is behind you?
- Where is the ball going? *(over my head)*
- Where are your arms? *(up high, up in the air)*
- What color is the ball?

When the ball reaches the last child, have him pass it to the other therapist who then leads the group in a final cheer of "1, 2, 3, Hurray!" Have the children elongate their trunks again as they raise their arms for the cheer.

Repeat the activity two or three times, depending on how well the children are paying attention.

Variations
1. Change the size, texture, and/or weight of the ball.
2. Change the children's body positions (e.g., sitting, standing, kneeling).

Activity 1: Monkey Swing

Have the children sit on a carpeted area or around a therapy mat. Explain that the children are going to pretend to be monkeys swinging from a tree branch. A broom handle will serve as the tree branch.

Have the other therapist hold one end of the broom while you hold the other so the handle is horizontally at a level that will require the children to extend their arms up. Call up one of the more capable children and have him face his peers. Instruct the child to reach up and hold onto the middle of the broom handle. Tell the child to lift his feet and "swing like a monkey," while you simultaneously raise the bar a few inches off of the ground. Have the other children count to 10 (can be reduced, if necessary) as the child swings. Let each child take a turn "swinging like a monkey."

Language prompts:
- Are you a monkey?
- What are you doing? *(swinging)*
- What does a monkey say?
- Where do monkeys live? *(jungle, zoo)*
- What do monkeys eat? *(bananas, fruit)*
- Do you like monkeys?
- Who has seen a real monkey?

Activity 2: Scooter Board Pull

Demonstrate a prone position on a scooter board. Maintain your legs and arms in extension with your head erect and neck extended. Have the other therapist show how to use a hula hoop to pull you across the room. The other therapist does this by slowly

walking backward while grasping the
hula hoop on one side with both hands
(bilateral hold) while you place both
hands on the hula hoop on the other
side with your arms extended. Have
her pull you across the room.

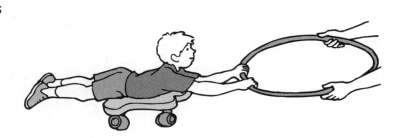

Then let the children take turns pulling
each other across the room. Make
sure each child gets a turn to pull and
be pulled on the scooter board.

Language prompts:
- What color is the scooter board?
- Point to the wheels. What are these called?
- How many wheels are there? *(four)*
- What are you holding? *(hula hoop)*
- What shape is the hoop? *(circle, round)*
- Who is pulling you?
- Who are you pulling?
- Are you walking backward?
- Are you lying on your back?
- Are you lying on your belly?

Variations
1. Have a child pull the scooter board in a side-stepping pattern, holding on to the hula
   hoop with one hand.
2. If you have two scooter boards and two hula hoops, this activity can be run as a race.

Activity 3: Pinwheel Game

Have the children return to their chairs. Show the children a pinwheel and demonstrate
how to take a deep breath and make the pinwheel spin as you release the air. Give each
child a turn to blow the pinwheel as you position it sideways in front of his mouth.

Language prompts:
- Refer to the pinwheel. What is this?
- Is the pinwheel big or little?
- Did you make your pinwheel move?
- Did you take a deep breath?

Variations
1. Move the pinwheel farther away from the child's mouth.
2. Change the size of the pinwheel. A smaller pinwheel requires a more forceful burst
   of air to make it spin.

Activity 4: Ghost Blow*

Have the children practice blowing into their hands so they can feel the air movement. Then show the children the ghost. Demonstrate how to make the ghost "fly" by blowing it as you suspend it in front of your face. Then carry the ghost around the circle of children so that each one can have several tries to blow and make the ghost move.

Language prompts:
- Did you feel the air?
- Refer to the ghost. What is this?
- What color is the ghost?
- Did you make the ghost fly?

Wrap-Up: Reintroduce the bee puppet to end the group, say good-bye to the children, and direct them to the next classroom activity.

> *Therapist:*   *"We're all finished! Let's say good-bye to Buzzy. Now it's time for (name of next classroom activity)."*

The classroom teacher then gives the children instructions about the next activity.

*Thanks to Barbara Parsons Davis, M.A., M.Ed., CCC-SLP, for the Ghost Blow activity.

Extra Activities

Extra activities can be used to reinforce October's themes and to lengthen the sessions if needed. Here are a few ideas to get you started.

Speech	OT
Breath Support	**Trunk Elongation**
• blowing feathers or leaves of various sizes	• *Bug and Worm Race*—Have the children crawl in quadruped like bugs and then switch to a commando crawl (facilitating elongation) to crawl like a worm.
• blowing party blowers	
• blowing whistles	• *Songs*—Have the group sing songs that encourage arms to be fully raised, such as *Itsy Bitsy Spider* and *Twinkle, Twinkle Little Star.**
• blowing out birthday candles	
• blowing paper towels to increase challenge (they are stiffer than tissues)	• *Basketball*—Have the children use a playground ball to shoot baskets into a hoop or box that is positioned to require bilateral arm extension.

*Hand/arm motions for *Twinkle, Twinkle Little Star*

Twinkle, twinkle little star	raise arms up in front of you and wiggle your fingers
How I wonder what you are.	
Up above the world so high	raise your arms, point your index fingers, and move your arms up and down
Like a diamond in the sky	make a diamond shape using both hands with your hands extended in front of your body and then above your head
Twinkle, twinkle little star	raise arms up in front of you and wiggle your fingers
How I wonder what you are!	

You can also make star wands by taping construction paper stars to the ends of straws. Have the children wave the stars and raise their arms as high as possible while singing the song.

Copyright © 2004 LinguiSystems, Inc.

NOVEMBER

Themes: Jaw Stabilization
Postural Control

Rationale

Speech: Jaw stabilization activities will help to promote movements that are independent from the head and tongue. A stable jaw is needed to produce a rapid sequence of phonemes which are necessary for typical speech production.

OT: Postural control and trunk stability are key to the development of a stable base from which to produce controlled distal hand function.

Helpful Hints:

 Keep Buzzy Bee within arm's reach so you can quickly access it during activities as needed.

 If behavior or attention is a problem, you may want to divide the children into two separate groups (or two lines, depending on the activity) to achieve more control of the group.

Materials: Buzzy Bee
small tray with handles
objects or pictures for tray (e.g., play food, box)
two cube chairs (cube chair has a back and a seat, but no legs)
chewy treats (e.g., gummy candy, fruit snacks)

Greeting: Have Buzzy Bee greet each child individually by saying, "Hi, (child's name)."   Encourage each child to respond appropriately to the puppet with verbal or nonverbal language.

> *Therapist:*   *"It's time to say hello to Buzzy Bee! Hi, Kelci!"*
> *Verbal Child:*   *"Hi, Buzzy!"*
>
> *Therapist:*   *"It's time to say hello to Buzzy Bee! Hi, Maria!"*
> *Nonverbal Child:* *Child must initiate eye contact and wave or smile.*

Warm-Up Activity: Have the children sit in two equal lines that face each other with a large floor space between them. Hand a small tray with handles to the child seated in the first chair. Put an object like a piece of play food or a small box on the tray. (You might want to use theme-related materials that correspond to the classroom curriculum.) Have the child hold the tray with both hands on the handles and walk carefully across the floor to the child opposite her without letting the object fall off of the tray. When the first child reaches the second child, the tray is passed to the second child. The second child then carries the tray across the room to the next child in line, and so on, until everyone has had a turn. Have the last child walk the tray back to a therapist to complete the activity.

Language prompts:
- Who is sitting next to you?
- Who is sitting across from you?
- Who has the tray?
- What is on the tray?

Variations
1. Use flat, stable objects or photographs of objects taped on the tray to decrease the level of challenge.
2. Increase the weight on the tray to increase the level of challenge.

Activity 1: Row Your Boat

Demonstrate how to sit on the floor with the other therapist. Sit facing each other with your legs in a V-shape. Place your lower legs/feet over the other therapists's lower legs. Hold hands. Show the children how to pull each other from a supine position (lying on back) to sitting while singing the song *Row, Row, Row Your Boat*. Then have the children get in pairs and sing the song. Repeat the song several times using varying speeds.

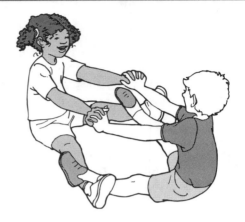

Activity 2: Cube Race

Have the children sit on the floor while both therapists demonstrate this activity. Get in a high kneel position (kneel with your bodies at a 90-degree angle) behind a cube chair. Race across the room, pushing the chairs, with your arms extended out straight in front of you.

Then have two children at a time race each other, using the same position. Be sure to have the children race in a section of the classroom or hallway that is carpeted. Put an object or tape on the floor about 10 feet away for the children to race to. Have the children who are watching provide verbal prompts (e.g., "Ready, Set, Go!").

Variations
1. Add weights or heavy books to the cube chairs to increase the level of challenge.
2. If cube chairs are not available, use boxes with heavy books in them.

Activity 3: Jaw Movements

Have the children sit on the floor with their backs against a wall and legs stretched out in front of them for postural stability. Since these jaw activities are more abstract than activities using manipulatives, introduce a chewy food reinforcer (e.g., gummy candy, fruit snacks) after each exercise. The food provides opportunities for more natural jaw movements.

1. Chewing: Model exaggerated chewing motions by moving your lower jaw up and down and side to side. Have the children imitate you and pretend to be cows.

2. "Ah": Demonstrate how to open your mouth and say "ah." Have the children open their mouths as if they were at the doctor's office. Remind the children to keep their heads erect. If their heads are tilted backward or forward, provide stabilization

through the use of physical prompts (e.g., apply light pressure to the top of the child's head with your right hand and under the child's chin with your left hand to assist the child in moving her head to the desired [erect] position).

3. Jaw Drop: Demonstrate how to perform a jaw drop by placing your fingers along your jaw line with your thumbs under your chin. Model how to drop your jaw with a verbal prompt (e.g., "Open your mouth wide"). Have the children feel their jaws drop by feeling the pressure against their thumbs. Repeat this activity five times. Look for chins jutting forward or moving laterally as this prevents the child from achieving proper jaw placement.

Wrap-Up: Reintroduce the bee puppet to end the group, say good-bye to the children, and direct them to the next classroom activity.

> *Therapist:* *"We're all finished! Let's say good-bye to Buzzy.*
> *Now it's time for (name of next classroom activity)."*

The classroom teacher then gives the children instructions about the next activity.

Copyright © 2004 LinguiSystems, Inc.

Materials: Buzzy Bee
small tray with handles
objects or pictures for tray (e.g., play food, box)
four (or more) coffee cans with plastic lids
variety of objects of varying weights and dimensions (e.g., pennies,
   marshmallows, blocks, jelly beans)
mirror
Goldfish crackers
plastic gloves (non-latex)

Greeting: Have Buzzy Bee greet each child individually by saying, "Hi, (child's name)."   Encourage each child to respond appropriately to the puppet with verbal or nonverbal language.

> *Therapist:*   "It's time to say hello to Buzzy Bee! Hi, Kelci!"
> *Verbal Child:*   "Hi, Buzzy!"

> *Therapist:*   "It's time to say hello to Buzzy Bee! Hi, Maria!"
> *Nonverbal Child:* Child must initiate eye contact and wave or smile.

Warm-Up Activity: Have the children sit in two equal lines that face each other with a large floor space between them. Hand a small tray with handles to the child seated in the first chair. Put an object like a piece of play food or a small box on the tray. (You might want to use theme-related materials that correspond to the classroom curriculum.) Have the child hold the tray with both hands on the handles and walk carefully across the floor to the child opposite her without letting the object fall off of the tray. When the first child reaches the second child, the tray is passed to the second child. The second child then carries the tray across the room to the next child in line, and so on, until everyone has had a turn. Have the last child walk the tray back to a therapist to complete the activity.

Language prompts:
- Who is sitting next to you?
- Who is sitting across from you?
- Who has the tray?
- What is on the tray?

Variations
1.   Use flat, stable objects or photographs of objects taped on the tray to decrease the level of challenge.
2.   Increase the weight on the tray to increase the level of challenge.

Activity 1: Crawling Race

Have the children sit on the floor to watch both therapists demonstrate a crawling race. Start in a quadruped (on all fours) position and crawl across the room, making sure to keep hands fully opened and to maintain an alternating bilateral pattern. Then have the children take turns racing each other using the same position to a target that is about 10 feet away. Be sure to have the children race in a section of the classroom or hallway that is carpeted. Have the children who are watching provide verbal prompts (e.g., "Ready, Set, Go!").

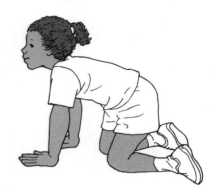

Variation: Repeat the activity with a beanbag placed on each child's back for additional sensory input.

Activity 2: Coffee Can Shake

Before the activity, place a generous handful of the pennies, marshmallows, etc. in each of the coffee cans. There should only be one type of object per can. Do not mix the items.

Have the children sit in their chairs in a circle. Place the coffee cans on the floor in the center of the circle. Demonstrate how to pick up a coffee can with two hands and lift it up to chest level. Then shake the can four or five times. Next lift your arms above your head and shake the can with your arms extended. Then move the can from one side of your body to the other, shaking the can two or three times on each side.

Have two children at a time pick up cans and shake them. Encourage each child to only move her arms to shake her can rather than move her whole body. Her body should remain stable. It may be necessary to help each child lift the can while keeping her feet stationary or to give a physical prompt at the child's hips to encourage trunk stability as the can is shaken. The children should not rotate their hips to face a different direction when shaking the can from side to side. They should reach across their bodies with the can, rotating their upper trunks from the waist up. (You might tell the children to shake the can by one ear and then the other to help them understand what to do.)

Encourage the children to listen and then guess what is in the cans as the cans are shaken.

After each child has shaken one can, have the children take turns opening the cans. You will need to put the lids back on to give each child a chance to open a can. When the cans are opened, beginning sounds can be reinforced. (See list on following page.)

- /m/ for marshmallow
- /p/ for pennies
- /b/ for blocks
- /k/ for can

At the end of the activity, give each child a jelly bean to eat. The chewy texture promotes rotary jaw movement and helps ready the children for the following oral motor activity.

Language prompts:
- Shake the can down low.
- Shake the can up high.
- Shake the can on this side.
- Shake the can on that side.
- What do you think is inside the can?
- Is the can heavy or light?

Variation: Change the weight of the objects in the cans.

Activity 3: Fish Face

Have the children sit with their legs extended and their heads and backs against the wall. Body position should be erect with a 90-degree angle at the hips for stability. Demonstrate how to open and close your mouth using slow and fast motions. Keep your head stationary against the wall, making sure your jaw movement is isolated.

Demonstrate a "fish face" (i.e., lip protrusion with a stable jaw). Then tell the children that they are going to pretend to be fish. Have them make fish faces. If a child cannot imitate this mouth posture, gently squeeze the child's cheeks to achieve lip protrusion. Make the fish face, release it, and count "1-2-3" five times. This will allow the children to practice while maintaining a slow pace. If you move too fast, it promotes movement of the head instead of movement of the jaw only.

Once the children have completed making the "fish face," have them be "singing fish" by singing "/ah/" and maintaining it for five seconds. If needed, an analogy can be made about a doctor fish telling a baby fish to open wide and say "/ah/."

Last, give each child a goldfish cracker. Encourage the children to hold them with their lips while maintaining a closed mouth position. If a child can't hold the cracker, you will see her chin drop. A light touch can be provided under the child's chin to assist with lip closure and a closed mouth. When the activity is over, reward the children verbally and by letting them eat the crackers.

Copyright © 2004 LinguiSystems, Inc.

Helpful Hints:

 If the child maintains an open mouth posture, it is helpful to allow the child to stabilize her jaw by placing her jaw on a table for extra support while maintaining a kneeling position.

 If the child cannot move her jaw independently of head movement, use a mirror to have the child watch herself.

Wrap-Up: Reintroduce the bee puppet to end the group, say good-bye to the children, and direct them to the next classroom activity.

> *Therapist:*   *"We're all finished! Let's say good-bye to Buzzy.*
> *Now it's time for (name of next classroom activity)."*

The classroom teacher then gives the children instructions about the next activity.

Week Three

Materials: Buzzy Bee
small tray with handles
objects or pictures for tray (e.g., play food, box)
play parachute or large sheet or blanket
chewy treats (e.g., gummy candy, fruit snacks, jelly beans)

Greeting: Have Buzzy Bee greet each child individually by saying, "Hi, (child's name)."   Encourage each child to respond appropriately to the puppet with verbal or nonverbal language.

> *Therapist:*   *"It's time to say hello to Buzzy Bee! Hi, Kelci!"*
> *Verbal Child:*   *"Hi, Buzzy!"*
>
> *Therapist:*   *"It's time to say hello to Buzzy Bee! Hi, Maria!"*
> *Nonverbal Child:* *Child must initiate eye contact and wave or smile.*

Warm-Up Activity: Have the children sit in two equal lines that face each other with a large floor space between them. Hand a small tray with handles to the child seated in the first chair. Put an object like a piece of play food or a small box on the tray. (You might want to use theme-related materials that correspond to the classroom curriculum.) Have the child hold the tray with both hands on the handles and walk carefully across the floor to the child opposite her without letting the object fall off of the tray. When the first child reaches the second child, the tray is passed to the second child. The second child then carries the tray across the room to the next child in line, and so on, until everyone has had a turn. Have the last child walk the tray back to a therapist to complete the activity.

Language prompts:
- Who is sitting next to you?
- Who is sitting across from you?
- Who has the tray?
- What is on the tray?

Variations
1. Use flat, stable objects or photographs of objects taped on the tray to decrease the level of challenge.
2. Increase the weight on the tray to increase the level of challenge.

Activity 1: Parachute*

Have the children take turns sitting in the middle of a play parachute while you and several of the other children pull it around the room or up and down a hallway. Make sure each child gets a turn to pull and to be pulled in the parachute.

Then play other parachute games such as "Ring-Around-the Rosy" and making a parachute "tent."

Activity 2: Silly Mouth Postures

Have the children sit with their legs extended and their heads and backs against the wall. Body position should be erect with a 90-degree angle at the hips for stability.

Demonstrate how to open and close your mouth using slow and fast motions. Keep your head stationary against the wall, making sure the jaw movement is isolated.

Have the children say, "Ah" and maintain it for five seconds. If needed, an analogy can be made about a doctor telling a child to open wide and say, "Ah."

Then give each child a small chewy treat. Remind the children to chew the treats while maintaining head stability. Give the children additional pieces as needed to practice independent jaw movements.

Wrap-Up: Reintroduce the bee puppet to end the group, say good-bye to the children, and direct them to the next classroom activity.

Therapist: "We're all finished! Let's say good-bye to Buzzy. Now it's time for (name of next classroom activity)."

The classroom teacher then gives the children instructions about the next activity.

*Since this activity is lengthy, it is the only sensory motor activity for this week.

Week Four

Materials:　Buzzy Bee
small tray with handles
objects or pictures for tray (e.g., play food, box)
medium-sized (18"–22") therapy ball
child-sized backpack
several cans of food
portable clinic stairs or other set of three stairs in the building
licorice sticks (two different colors/flavors, one per child and therapist)
plastic gloves (non-latex)

Greeting:　Have Buzzy Bee greet each child individually by saying, "Hi, (child's name)."　Encourage each child to respond appropriately to the puppet with verbal or nonverbal language.

> *Therapist:*　　　*"It's time to say hello to Buzzy Bee!　Hi, Kelci!"*
> *Verbal Child:*　　*"Hi, Buzzy!"*
>
> *Therapist:*　　　*"It's time to say hello to Buzzy Bee!　Hi, Maria!"*
> *Nonverbal Child:*　*Child must initiate eye contact and wave or smile.*

Warm-Up Activity:　Have the children sit in two equal lines that face each other with a large floor space between them.　Hand a small tray with handles to the child seated in the first chair.　Put an object like a piece of play food or a small box on the tray.　(You might want to use theme-related materials that correspond to the classroom curriculum.)　Have the child hold the tray with both hands on the handles and walk carefully across the floor to the child opposite her without letting the object fall off of the tray.　When the first child reaches the second child, the tray is passed to the second child.　The second child then carries the tray across the room to the next child in line, and so on, until everyone has had a turn.　Have the last child walk the tray back to a therapist to complete the activity.

Language prompts:
- Who is sitting next to you?
- Who is sitting across from you?
- Who has the tray?
- What is on the tray?

Variations
1. Use flat, stable objects or photographs of objects taped on the tray to decrease the level of challenge.
2. Increase the weight on the tray to increase the level of challenge.

Activity 1: Ball Rides

Show the children the therapy ball. Explain that each child will have a turn to get a "tummy ride" on the ball. Invite one child to demonstrate. Position the child prone over the ball. Keep your hands on the child's hips at all times. Explain that you want her to "walk" forward on her hands while you stabilize her hips and lower extremities. Have the other therapist sit about three feet away. Tell the child to give the other therapist a "high-five" sign when she reaches her. Then with your grasp firmly maintained on the child's hips, pull her back to her starting point, giving her a "ride" on the ball. (Note: The child should always have part of her body on the ball.) Give each child a turn.

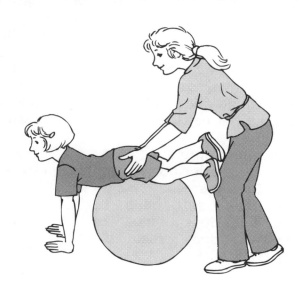

Activity 2: Backpack Picnic

Have the children sit down. Explain that they are going to pretend to go on a picnic. Show them the backpack and the cans of food they will take.

Have one child come up and choose a can. Help her put the can in the backpack and then put the backpack on her back. Have her walk up three therapy stairs and down again to a pretend picnic area. Have the other therapist greet her and remove the backpack so that the next child can have a turn.

Variations
1. Have the more capable children walk up and down the stairs with more than one can of food in the backpack.
2. For children who cannot manage a backpack on stairs, put a line of masking tape on the floor several feet away. Have the child walk to the line and back again. The tape serves as a visual prompt for the child.

Activity 3: Licorice Pull

Have the children sit in chairs with their backs up against the backs of the chairs. Sitting in a chair, cup your hands and place them under the chair seat, one hand on each side of the seat. Have the children place their hands the same way. Then demonstrate how to tense your body while pulling up/holding on to the chair seat. By tensing your body, you are forced to clench your teeth without much effort. Have the children tense their bodies the same way. Repeat this at least three times.

Copyright © 2004 LinguiSystems, Inc.

Week Four, *continued*

Once the children have practiced this, put on the plastic gloves and get one piece of licorice. Place the piece horizontally in the other therapist's mouth on her molars and have her bite down lightly on the licorice. Then have her pull the licorice toward the front of her mouth while holding onto the right and left sides of the licorice.

Now do this activity with each child. Show the child the two colors/flavors of licorice and let her choose one. Place the licorice in her mouth and have her lightly bite down. (The child should not bite through the licorice.) Repeat two or three times. After the child's turn, let her eat the licorice as a reward.

Language prompts:
- What color do you want? *(I want red licorice. I want brown licorice.)*
- Does it smell?
- Does it smell good?
- What does it smell like?
- What does it feel like?
- Is it sticky?

Wrap-Up: Reintroduce the bee puppet to end the group, say good-bye to the children, and direct them to the next classroom activity.

> *Therapist:*   *"We're all finished! Let's say good-bye to Buzzy.*
> *Now it's time for (name of next classroom activity)."*

The classroom teacher then gives the children instructions about the next activity.

Use extra activities to reinforce November's themes and to lengthen the sessions if needed. Here are a few ideas to get you started.

Speech
Jaw Stabilization

- Instead of a licorice pull, try using a pretzel rod, tongue depressor, or Popsicle stick.

- Bite a chewy food (e.g., gummy candy, shoestring licorice tied into a small knot) with your incisors while someone else pulls on the food item.

- Chew crunchy food items (e.g., apples, pears).

- Chew various types of crackers (e.g., Ritz, Saltines).

- Chew various types of cookies (e.g., chocolate chip, Oreos).

OT
Postural Control

- Play wheelbarrow walk games. Have the child put her hands on the floor in a prone position while a therapist or another child holds the child's legs between the knees and the ankles. The child "walks" forward like a wheelbarrow.

- Pull a toy wagon with items of varying weights in it.

- Do wall push-ups (pretend to "push" the wall). Depending on the child's height, have her stand a step or two away from the wall. Have her place her arms straight in front of her and put her hands flat on the wall. To do the wall push-up, she should bend her elbows to shift her body forward. Then she should straighten her arms to move her body back to its initial position. Repeat a few times, depending on the child's strength and ability.

- Push toy cars along a masking tape line on the floor while crawling next to the line.

- Have a tug-of-war with a heavy rope.

Copyright © 2004 LinguiSystems, Inc.

DECEMBER

Theme: Review

Due to winter vacation, December is designated as a review month. Choose your favorite activities from October and November and/or supplement with the October or November extra activity ideas. Make sure to include the Greeting, a Warm-Up Activity, and the Wrap-Up.

JANUARY

Themes: Lip Closure

Wrist Control

Rationale

Speech: Lip closure activities will help strengthen the lip muscles so they remain closed in the child's natural resting position. Lip closure is essential for the production of /p, b/, and /m/ in words, phrases, sentences, and conversational speech.

OT: Wrist control is fundamental for the development of functional hand skills. The wrist is usually in slight extension and supination when using most tools (e.g., crayons, scissors). Therefore, it is crucial that children learn to position their wrists in extension, supination, and pronation, and be able to transition between these positions.

Helpful Hints: Keep Buzzy Bee within arm's reach so you can quickly access it during activities as needed.

 If behavior or attention is a problem, you may want to divide the children into two separate groups (or two lines, depending on the activity) to achieve more control of the group.

Materials: Buzzy Bee
three bathroom-sized paper cups
three stickers (put one on the bottom inside surface of each paper
    cup before the activity)
tongue depressors or plastic straws (one per child and therapist)
2½" x ½" pretzel dipping sticks (one per child and therapist)

(Note: The pretzel dipping sticks are for the third activity. Do not use thin pretzel sticks or pretzel rods. Pretzel dipping sticks are also called *stix, old-fashioned sticks,* or *pennysticks*.)

Greeting: Have Buzzy Bee greet each child individually by saying, "Hi, (child's name)." Encourage each child to respond appropriately to the puppet with verbal or nonverbal language.

> *Therapist:*   "*It's time to say hello to Buzzy Bee! Hi, Evan!*"
> *Verbal Child:*   "*Hi, Buzzy!*"
>
> *Therapist:*   "*It's time to say hello to Buzzy Bee! Hi, Jamal!*"
> *Nonverbal Child:* *Child must initiate eye contact and wave or smile.*

Warm-Up Activity: Have the children sit in chairs or on the floor. Sit facing the other therapist. Each of you should hold your hands in front of your body with your arms slightly flexed (bent) at the elbows to demonstrate the hand-clapping pattern. (Your hands should be vertical.) Touch your hands to the other therapist's hands in pronation (palms of hands), then in supination (back of hands), and then back to pronation. Model a three-word phrase (e.g., "I like snow") as you touch your hands together. Verbalize one word with each hand motion. Then have each child do this activity with each therapist, getting two turns to practice the motions. Vary the phrase to correspond to the classroom curriculum (e.g., snow theme—"I like snow," food theme—"apples and bananas").

Variation: Have the children attempt this task with each other.

Copyright © 2004 LinguiSystems, Inc.

Activity 1: Charades

Have the children sit in a row or a semicircle. Lead the children in the song, "This is the way we brush our hair" while acting out the motion of hair brushing. Choose pantomimes that facilitate wrist movements (e.g., hand washing, hair brushing, tooth brushing, opening a door/turning the knob, waving, and turning a key). Change the song lyrics to reflect the motion.

Activity 2: Hidden Stickers

Have the children remain seated. Place three small bathroom cups (with stickers inside) upside down on a flat surface. Demonstrate how to crawl to the cups. Be sure to promote wrist extension and shoulder stability. Then grasp and turn over each cup to view the sticker inside. After looking at the sticker in the cup, put the cup back in its place. Have each child take a turn crawling up to look into the cups. You might want to use stickers that correspond to the classroom curriculum (e.g., animals, fruit) or use stickers that have pictures of things starting with /p, b/, and /m/.

Language prompts:
- What sticker do you see inside the cup?
- What color is the sticker?
- Did your lips touch? (when child produces the target sound)

Activity 3: Lip Games

Have the children continue to sit in a row or a semicircle. Give one tongue depressor or straw to each child. Close your lips and demonstrate how to "wake up" your lips by tapping them with the tongue depressor. Have each child "wake up" his lips in the same way. Give verbal prompts as needed if a child's lips are not closed (e.g., "Put your lips together, make your lips touch, hide your teeth.").

Then have each child take a turn holding a tongue depressor horizontally in his lips (not his teeth) for a count of 5 and then release it into your hand.

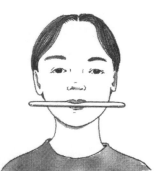

After three turns with the tongue depressor (i.e., taking the tongue depressor out of the child's mouth and then putting it back in), throw the tongue depressor away.

Then pass out the pretzel dipping sticks. Have the children hold the pretzel horizontally with their lips and not with their teeth. It may be helpful to introduce the imagery of a dog holding his bone for those children having difficulty. Once the child has held the pretzel for a designated amount of time (length of time depends on the child's ability to hold the pretzel), let the child eat the pretzel.

Copyright © 2004 LinguiSystems, Inc.

Week One, *continued*

Variation: Have the children follow one-step hand movements while holding the tongue depressor or pretzel with their lips. The movements can be in the form of a "Simon Says" game and should be chosen to facilitate wrist motions (e.g., turn a knob, wave good-bye, touch your back).

Wrap-Up: Reintroduce the bee puppet to end the group, say good-bye to the children, and direct them to the next classroom activity.

> *Therapist:* "We're all finished! Let's say good-bye to Buzzy. Now it's time for (name of next classroom activity)."

The classroom teacher then gives the children instructions about the next activity.

Materials: Buzzy Bee
pairs of animal flash cards
shaker for each child (empty toilet paper roll, uncooked macaroni inside, clear packing tape)
colorful stickers (one for each shaker)
straws (one per child and therapist)
Froot Loops (three per child and therapist)
party blowers (one per child)
small plastic zippered bags
black permanent marker (for labeling blowers/bags)

(Note: The shaker is for the second activity. To make a shaker, securely cover one end of the toilet paper roll with tape. Put some uncooked macaroni in the tube and securely cover the other end with tape so the macaroni will not fall out. Put a sticker on one end of the shaker.)

Greeting: Have Buzzy Bee greet each child individually by saying, "Hi, (child's name)." Encourage each child to respond appropriately to the puppet with verbal or nonverbal language.

Therapist:	*"It's time to say hello to Buzzy Bee! Hi, Evan!"*
Verbal Child:	*"Hi, Buzzy!"*

Therapist:	*"It's time to say hello to Buzzy Bee! Hi, Jamal!"*
Nonverbal Child:	*Child must initiate eye contact and wave or smile.*

Warm-Up Activity: Have the children sit in chairs or on the floor. Sit facing the other therapist. Each of you should hold your hands in front of your body with your arms slightly flexed (bent) at the elbows to demonstrate the hand-clapping pattern. (Your hands should be vertical.) Touch your hands to the other therapist's hands in pronation (palms of hands), then in supination (back of hands), and then back to pronation. Model a three-word phrase (e.g., "I like snow") as you touch your hands together. Verbalize one word with each hand motion. Then have each child do this activity with each therapist, getting two turns to practice the motions. Vary the phrase to correspond to the classroom curriculum (e.g., snow theme—"I like snow," food theme—"apples and bananas").

Variation: Have the children attempt this task with each other.

Week Two, *continued*

Activity 1: Animal Hunt

Have the children sit in chairs or on the floor. Place the flash cards or picture cards faceup in pairs on the floor away from the children. For lower-functioning children, put the pairs right next to each other. For higher-functioning children, mix up the cards.

Have each child crawl across the floor with hands fully extended to the flash cards. Instruct each child to find specific cards using a verbal prompt such as "Find the two elephants." The child then uses his dominant hand to turn over the matching cards one at a time (i.e., "hiding" the pictures). Then have the child crawl back to his seat.

Language prompts:
- What animal is on the card that you turned over?
- What does the animal say?
- Is the animal big or small?

Activity 2: Macaroni Shakers

Have the children remain seated on the floor. Give each child a shaker. Demonstrate how to shake the shaker, using a stable shoulder and forearm with only your wrist providing the motion. Have the children imitate this movement and other movements such as shaking the shaker by each ear, shaking the shaker high and low, and shaking with a wrist-flipping movement (pronation and supination). Then have the children stand their shakers upright with the stickers showing on the top. Have the children turn the shakers over to hide the stickers. Repeat several times so the children can practice pronating and supinating their wrists as they turn the shakers.

Activity 3: Froot Loop Pull

Before this activity, place three Froot Loops on a straw for each child.

Have the children remain seated. Hum so the children can hear you. Then have each child hum. Make sure lip closure is achieved. If humming is performed correctly, the child will be able to feel the vibration on his nose by placing his index finger on the side of his nose. When each child has achieved lip closure, continue with this activity.

Demonstrate how to pull one Froot Loop at a time off of a straw with your lips. Eat each Froot Loop as you pull it off. Then hold a straw for the first child while he pulls the Froot Loops, one at a time, off the straw. Do the same for each child, using a new straw each time.

Copyright © 2004 LinguiSystems, Inc.

Activity 4: Party Blowers

Give each child a party blower. Have each child manually uncurl the blower with his hands several times. This will help the blower be less stiff and it promotes wrist mobility. Then have each child take a deep breath and blow into the blower while maintaining lip closure. Encourage the children to blow into the blower several times. For more fun, have the children sit in a circle and blow the party blowers at one another.

(Note: Store the blowers in plastic zippered bags. Label each bag with the child's name so the blowers don't get mixed up and can be used at a later time. If possible, label the blowers too.)

Variation: Have the children assume a high kneel position to promote breath support and trunk elongation.

Wrap-Up: Reintroduce the bee puppet to end the group, say good-bye to the children, and direct them to the next classroom activity.

Therapist: *"We're all finished! Let's say good-bye to Buzzy. Now it's time for (name of next classroom activity)."*

The classroom teacher then gives the children instructions about the next activity.

57

Copyright © 2004 LinguiSystems, Inc.

Week Three

Materials: Buzzy Bee
hand lotion (hypoallergenic and non-scented)
animal stickers (two per child and extras)
hand puppets (at least four)
Cheerios (at least three per child and therapist)
coffee stirrers (one per child and therapist)

Greeting: Have Buzzy Bee greet each child individually by saying, "Hi, (child's name)." Encourage each child to respond appropriately to the puppet with verbal or nonverbal language.

> *Therapist:* "It's time to say hello to Buzzy Bee! Hi, Evan!"
> *Verbal Child:* "Hi, Buzzy!"
>
> *Therapist:* "It's time to say hello to Buzzy Bee! Hi, Jamal!"
> *Nonverbal Child:* Child must initiate eye contact and wave or smile.

Warm-Up Activity: Have the children sit in chairs or on the floor. Sit facing the other therapist. Each of you should hold your hands in front of your body with your arms slightly flexed (bent) at the elbows to demonstrate the hand-clapping pattern. (Your hands should be vertical.) Touch your hands to the other therapist's hands in pronation (palms of hands), then in supination (back of hands), and then back to pronation. Model a three-word phrase (e.g., "I like snow") as you touch your hands together. Verbalize one word with each hand motion. Then have each child do this activity with each therapist, getting two turns to practice the motions. Vary the phrase to correspond to the classroom curriculum (e.g., snow theme—"I like snow," food theme—"apples and bananas").

Variation: Have the children attempt this task with each other.

Activity 1: Lotion

Have the children sit on the floor. Put a small amount of lotion on the dorsal (back) side of your hand. Demonstrate how to rotate your wrists to spread the lotion on all of your hand surfaces. Then put a small amount of hand lotion on the dorsal (back) side of each child's hands and have the children practice this activity. Some physical prompts may be necessary to achieve wrist rotation (e.g., touch the back of the child's hand that doesn't have lotion on it as you say "Don't forget to put it here"). Some children may need hand-over-hand assistance to get started with the motion.

Activity 2: Animal Sticker Game

Place two different animal stickers on the dorsal sides of each child's hands. Explain to the children that you are the farmer in charge of the animals. Have the children place their hands palm side down on the carpet with the stickers showing. Explain that it is time for the animals to "go to sleep" (i.e., have the children turn their hands to a palm-up position so the stickers are not visible). Then have the animals to "wake up" (i.e., have the children turn their hands palm down so the stickers are visible). Repeat several times.

Language prompts:
- What animals are on your hands?
- What does the animal say?
- Are your animals asleep?
- Are your animals awake?

Variation: Explain to the children that only one animal needs to go to sleep. Demonstrate how to supinate (turn over) one hand instead of two. Have the children practice several times, varying which hand is turned over.

Activity 3: Puppets

Give each child a hand puppet. If there are not enough puppets available, have the children take turns. Use Buzzy Bee to lead them through a number of different motions that facilitate wrist control and mobility, including the following.

- making the puppet "dance" by rotating your wrist
- making the puppet bow
- making the puppet lie down on the carpet to "sleep," "roll over," and then "wake up"

Week Three, *continued*

Language prompts:
- Which puppet do you want?
- Which puppet did you choose?
- What color is your puppet?
- Who has (name of puppet)?
- Which puppet does (name of child) have?

Activity 4: Cheerio Pull

Before this activity, place three Cheerios on one coffee stirrer for each child.

Demonstrate how to open and close your mouth while smacking your lips together to make a popping sound. (Some children do not know where their lips are located or they have an open mouth posture, so this will provide stimulation of the lips and get them ready for the next part of the activity.)

Once the children can demonstrate the lip popping, show the children how to say "pah, pay," and "po." Then have the children say the syllables in repetition (e.g., "pah pah, pay pay, po po"). Encourage them to produce the syllables slowly and then quickly. Make sure lip closure is achieved as they practice. If a child is having difficulty achieving lip closure, have him repeat the syllables several times for more practice.

Demonstrate how to pull one Cheerio at a time off of a coffee stirrer with your lips. Eat each Cheerio as you pull it off. Then hold a coffee stirrer for the first child while he pulls the Cheerios, one at a time, off the coffee stirrer. Do the same for each child, using a new coffee stirrer each time.

Wrap-Up: Reintroduce the bee puppet to end the group, say good-bye to the children, and direct them to the next classroom activity.

> *Therapist:* "*We're all finished! Let's say good-bye to Buzzy. Now it's time for (name of next classroom activity).*"

The classroom teacher then gives the children instructions about the next activity.

                    Copyright © 2004 LinguiSystems, Inc.

Materials: Buzzy Bee
small windup toys of various sizes and types (one per child if possible)
empty spice containers (one per child; containers should be small, clean,
   plastic, and clear)
M&Ms
lip balm (e.g., Chapstick)
cotton swabs (one per child and therapist)
tongue depressors (one per child and therapist)
pennies (two per child and therapist)
tape

Greeting: Have Buzzy Bee greet each child individually by saying, "Hi, (child's
name)." Encourage each child to respond appropriately to the puppet
with verbal or nonverbal language.

> *Therapist:*   "*It's time to say hello to Buzzy Bee! Hi, Evan!*"
> *Verbal Child:*   "*Hi, Buzzy!*"

> *Therapist:*   "*It's time to say hello to Buzzy Bee! Hi, Jamal!*"
> *Nonverbal Child:* *Child must initiate eye contact and wave or smile.*

Warm-Up
Activity: Have the children sit in chairs or on the floor. Sit facing the other
therapist. Each of you should hold your hands in front of your body with
your arms slightly flexed (bent) at the elbows to demonstrate the hand-
clapping pattern. (Your hands should be vertical.) Touch your hands to
the other therapist's hands in pronation (palms of hands), then in
supination (back of hands), and then back to pronation. Model a three-
word phrase (e.g., "I like snow") as you touch your hands together.
Verbalize one word with each hand motion. Then have each child do this
activity with each therapist, getting two turns to practice the motions.
Vary the phrase to correspond to the classroom curriculum (e.g., snow
theme—"I like snow," food theme—"apples and bananas").

Variation: Have the children attempt this task with each other.

Activity 1: WindUp Toys

Bring out the windup toys. Demonstrate how to use your thumb, index finger, and middle finger to grasp the knob on a toy and wind it three times. Place the toy on the floor to watch it move. Then give each child a windup toy to practice winding. Let the children switch toys with each other to have more practice learning this skill.

(Note: This activity works best on a non-carpeted surface such as a tile floor or a table.)

Language prompts:
- Which toy do you have?
- Which toy does (name of child) have?
- Ask (name of child) for a toy.

Activity 2: Spice Jar Games

Before the activity, put one M&M in each spice jar. Then give a spice jar to each child. Demonstrate how to shake the jar up and down and side to side. Have the children imitate your movements while maintaining a stable trunk. Then have the children place their containers upside-down so the lid is on the floor. Have them practice turning the container several times so that the lid is up and then down. Be sure each child maintains a stable shoulder and trunk when turning the jars over.

When you are done, let the children unscrew the lids to get the candy. For more wrist rotation practice, put additional M&Ms in the jars.

Activity 3: Tongue Depressor Balance

Have the children sit against the wall on the floor with their legs stretched out in front of them for additional postural stability/support. Smear a dab of lip balm onto a cotton swab. Then spread the lip balm on your lips using the cotton swab. After you put the lip balm on your lips, close your lips and continue the oral stimulation by tapping your lips with the cotton swab. Then put lip balm on each child's lips, using a new cotton swab each time. Have the children practice humming for a few seconds to feel the lip vibration with the additional tactile stimulation of the lip balm. Encourage lip closure by having the children say the syllables "me, may," and "mah." Also have the children prolong the /m/ sound as well as reduplicate the syllables (e.g., "me me me, may may may, mah mah mah").

Have the children transition to chairs. Make sure the children are sitting with their backs up against the backs of the chairs. Sitting in a chair, cup your hands and place them under the chair seat, one hand on each side of the seat. Have the children place their hands the same way. Then demonstrate how to tense your body while pulling up/holding on to the chair seat. By tensing your body, you are forced to clench your teeth without much effort. Have the children tense their bodies the same way. Repeat this activity at least three times.

Once the children have practiced this activity, demonstrate how to hold a tongue depressor horizontally with only your lips in front of your central incisors. Do not use your teeth. Then give one tongue depressor to each child and have him hold it horizontally in his lips for various time increments (e.g., 5 seconds, 7 seconds, 10 seconds) without using his teeth.

When each child can hold the tongue depressor in his lips, tape one penny to each end of the tongue depressor. The pennies require the children to control their lips more by pressing their lips more firmly together. You might want to use flavored tongue depressors and have the children guess which flavor they are using.

Variations

1. Use Popsicle sticks to make the task easier. They are not as wide or as heavy as tongue depressors.
2. Have contests between the children. See which child can hold his tongue depressor the longest without dropping it.
3. Have contests between the children and therapists. See who can hold his tongue depressor the longest without dropping it. You might challenge the children by saying, "See if you can hold it longer than me."

Wrap-Up: Reintroduce the bee puppet to end the group, say good-bye to the children, and direct them to the next classroom activity.

> Therapist: *"We're all finished! Let's say good-bye to Buzzy.
> Now it's time for (name of next classroom activity)."*

The classroom teacher then gives the children instructions about the next activity.

Extra Activities

Use extra activities to reinforce January's themes and to lengthen the sessions if needed. Here are a few ideas to get you started.

Speech	OT
Lip Closure	**Wrist Control**

Speech

Lip Closure

- Play a snake game with your tongue. Have the child move his snake (tongue) in and out of his mouth slowly and quickly. Encourage him to maintain lip closure in between movements.

- Stroke the child's lips with a washcloth. Press the washcloth on the child's lips. Have the child hold the washcloth with his lips while you try to pull it out.

- Have the child brush his teeth. Then place the toothbrush in his mouth with the bristles touching his tongue and the handle pointing straight out of his mouth. Have the child hold the toothbrush in his mouth with his lips. Encourage lip closure for increasing intervals of time.

- Use a small lollipop (e.g., DumDum lollipops) to tap the child's lips and then slide it along his lips. Place the lollipop in the child's mouth to try to achieve lip closure. Say things like, "Hide your lollipop" or "Hold the lollipop with no hands." You can also have contests to see who can hold the lollipop in his mouth the longest.

- Have the child hold various food items with only his lips to achieve lip closure (e.g., crackers, licorice, potato chips).

- Have the child drink from cups or juice boxes with a straw as this promotes natural lip closure.

OT

Wrist Control

- Play games that require a child to turn over a sand timer (e.g., have the children complete a task before the sand runs out).

- Use a rain stick. The children will have fun turning the rain stick to hear the sounds it makes.

- Play with a Slinky. Make the Slinky move, holding one end with each hand.

- Play games with a beanbag, such as throwing the beanbag into targets.

- Have snacks that require spoon use (e.g., pudding, ice cream).

- Play games where the children have to open and close classroom doors or closets by turning a doorknob (e.g., hide-and-seek with stuffed animals).

- Practice pouring liquids from one container to another.

Copyright © 2004 LinguiSystems, Inc.

FEBRUARY

Themes: Tongue Elevation

Bilateral Motor Skills and Midline Crossing

Rationale

Speech: Tongue elevation activities will help strengthen the tip of the tongue. Tongue elevation is essential for the production of /t, d, n, s, l, z/ and /ch/ in words, phrases, sentences, and conversational speech.

OT: To develop a skillful dominant hand, children must be able to cross the midline of the body in activities. A well-established dominant hand is necessary to achieve fine motor control. The non-dominant hand is also important to stabilize objects as the dominant hand performs an activity. Therefore, children must acquire bilateral integration as well as midline crossing.

Helpful Hints:

 Keep Buzzy Bee within arm's reach so you can quickly access it during activities as needed.

 If behavior or attention is a problem, you may want to divide the children into two separate groups (or two lines, depending on the activity) to achieve more control of the group.

     Copyright © 2004 LinguiSystems, Inc.

Week One

Materials: Buzzy Bee
three drums (coffee cans with lids, foil)
long-handled spoons (wooden or plastic) or drumsticks
beanbags
bathroom-sized paper cups (one for each child and therapist)
plastic spoons (one for each child and therapist)
one container of thawed Cool Whip

(Note: The drums are for the first activity. To make a drum, cover a coffee can
with foil and place the lid on it.)

Greeting: Have Buzzy Bee greet each child individually by saying, "Hi, (child's
name)." Encourage each child to respond appropriately to the puppet
with verbal or nonverbal language.

> *Therapist:*   *"It's time to say hello to Buzzy Bee! Hi, Kelci!"*
> *Verbal Child:*   *"Hi, Buzzy!"*
>
> *Therapist:*   *"It's time to say hello to Buzzy Bee! Hi, Maria!"*
> *Nonverbal Child:* *Child must initiate eye contact and wave or smile.*

Warm-Up Activity: Have the children sit in chairs or on the floor. With the other therapist,
demonstrate a two-person hand-clapping pattern. Hold your hands in
front of your bodies with your palms facing each other. Touch hands.
Crisscross your hands and have your palms meet again. Then uncross
your hands and have your palms touch again. End the pattern with a
clap. Model a four-word phrase such as "One, two, three, magic" as you
touch, crisscross, uncross, and clap hands. Have each child do the
pattern with each therapist, thereby getting two turns to practice the
motions.

(Note: You might want the four-word phrase to reflect your classroom theme
[e.g., "pink hearts, red hearts"].)

Variation: Have the children attempt the hand-clapping pattern with
one another.

Activity 1: Beat the Drums

Part One: Have the children sit in a semicircle in their chairs. Place one drum in the center of the group. It may be helpful to have several beanbags in the can to maintain its stability. Explain to the children that your hands will "take turns" beating the drum with the drumsticks (e.g., long-handled spoons). Demonstrate how to "beat" the drum by holding a spoon in each hand and tapping the top of the can with them in an alternating bilateral pattern. Then have each child come up to beat the drum a number of times. The rest of the children can sing a rhythmic song to help mark the beat (e.g., the alphabet song) or have them practice at the same time by tapping their knees to the beat of a song using a bilateral motion (using both hands).

Part Two: Bring out two more coffee can drums and arrange them in an arc with the original drum. Using only one drumstick, hit the drum on the far left once and then hit the other drums in line, one time each. You might say a rhyme such as, "One, two, three, play the drums like me." Repeat the sequence. Then give each child a turn to hit the drums. Present the drumstick in the middle of the child's body. She will most likely use her dominant hand to hold the drumstick.

Language Prompts:
- Point to drum. What is this? *(drum, can)*
- What are you tapping/hitting?
- Who is tapping?
- Is the noise loud or soft?

Activity 2: Simon Says

Have the children sit in their chairs or on the floor. Lead the children in a game of Simon Says, emphasizing positions that promote bilateral coordination and midline crossing in the upper and lower body. Have the children imitate your motions as you say things like "Simon Says put your hands like this" (as you put both hands on your right hip) or "Simon Says move your legs like this" (as you cross and uncross your legs). Here are some examples you can demonstrate for the children to imitate:

- right hand on left shoulder
- wave arms above head in a crossing/uncrossing pattern
- left hand on right ear
- right hand on left knee
- right hand touching left elbow while left hand is touching right elbow

(Note: All of these activities can be reversed so the child must cross the midline using the other hand.)

Language Prompts:
- What did Simon say to do?
- Are your arms crossed or uncrossed?
- Where are your hands?
- What are you doing? *(playing a game, putting hands on hip, waving arms)*

Activity 3: Tongue Lift

Have the children transition to the floor with their heads and backs against the wall to achieve stabilization of the head and jaw. Demonstrate tongue elevation by attempting to reach your nose with your tongue. Then have the children try it. Remind the children to let their tongues do the work, not their heads or necks.

Verbal prompts might be helpful (e.g., "Pretend you have ice cream on your nose. Lick it off with your tongue."). Head and jaw stabilization may need to be assisted with physical prompts (e.g., hold the child's head with your hands on her cheeks or hold the child's head with one hand on top of her head and one under her chin).

Variation: Have the children kneel at a table. As a prompt, have them place their chins on the table so their heads cannot easily move forward or backward.

Activity 4: Cool Whip Lick

Have the children continue to sit on the floor. Put some thawed Cool Whip in a cup with a plastic spoon. Scoop some Cool Whip onto the spoon and hold it vertically in front of your mouth. Demonstrate how to use your tongue tip to lick the Cool Whip off the spoon. Then give one child at a time a spoon and a cup with a small amount of Cool Whip so she can practice lifting her tongue. The child may be able to hold the spoon herself, but you may need to assist the child by holding the spoon in the right position. Head and jaw must be stable to achieve desired tongue elevation. Don't allow the child to tilt her head backward or forward.

Language Prompts:
- What color is the Cool Whip?
- Is the Cool Whip soft or hard? Hot or cold?
- What are you doing with your tongue? *(licking the Cool Whip, lifting it)*
- Who likes to eat Cool Whip?

Activity 5: Friendship Circle

Have the children sit close together in chairs or on the floor in a circle. Show them how to cross their arms and hold hands with the children next to them on either side in a "Friendship Circle." Lead the children in a familiar, calming song such as "Twinkle, Twinkle Little Star" while they sway side to side, maintaining the crossed-hand link. After the song is completed, encourage the children to give themselves "hugs" with their arms crossing midline and wrapping around their bodies.

Language Prompts:
- Who is sitting next to you?
- What are you doing with your hands/arms? *(holding hands, crossing arms)*
- While singing the song, have the children fill in missing words (e.g., "Twinkle, Twinkle, _____ star").
- Whose hands are you holding?

Wrap-Up: Reintroduce the bee puppet to end the group, say good-bye to the children, and direct them to the next classroom activity.

> *Therapist:* "*We're all finished! Let's say good-bye to Buzzy. Now it's time for (name of next classroom activity)."*

The classroom teacher then gives the children instructions about the next activity.

Week Two

Materials: Buzzy Bee
several decorative stickers
six colorful beanbags
therapy barrel
package of sandwich cookies (e.g., Oreos, vanilla/chocolate)

Greeting: Have Buzzy Bee greet each child individually by saying, "Hi, (child's name)." Encourage each child to respond appropriately to the puppet with verbal or nonverbal language.

> *Therapist:*   *"It's time to say hello to Buzzy Bee! Hi, Kelci!"*
> *Verbal Child:*   *"Hi, Buzzy!"*
>
> *Therapist:*   *"It's time to say hello to Buzzy Bee! Hi, Maria!"*
> *Nonverbal Child:* *Child must initiate eye contact and wave or smile.*

Warm-Up Activity: Have the children sit in chairs or on the floor. With the other therapist, demonstrate a two-person hand-clapping pattern. Hold your hands in front of your bodies with your palms facing each other. Touch hands. Crisscross your hands and have your palms meet again. Then uncross your hands and have your palms touch again. End the pattern with a clap. Model a four-word phrase such as "One, two, three, magic" as you touch, crisscross, uncross, and clap hands. Have each child do the pattern with each therapist, thereby getting two turns to practice the motions.

(Note: You might want the four-word phrase to reflect your classroom theme [e.g., "pink hearts, red hearts"].)

Variation: Have the children attempt the hand-clapping pattern with one another.

Activity 1: Sticker Game

Have the children sit against a wall or in chairs in a circle. Invite one child up to demonstrate the activity. Place a decorative sticker lightly on the child's left shoulder. Gently hold the child's left hand to prevent its use. Have the child find the sticker. Encourage her to reach across her midline with her free right hand to retrieve the sticker. Repeat the activity several times with each child and vary it as suggested:

- Place the sticker on the left cheek. Retrieve with the right hand.
- Place the sticker on the right ear. Retrieve with the left hand.
- Place the sticker on the left side of the neck. Retrieve with the right hand.

Language prompts:
- Where is the sticker?
- Do you have the sticker?
- Who has the sticker?
- What is on your sticker?
- What color is your sticker?

Activity 2: Beanbag Game

Have two children at a time sit straddled over a barrel that is laid horizontally on the floor. The children should sit facing the same direction. Sit on the left side of the children and offer the beanbag to the child in the front. Have her reach for the beanbag across her midline (using her right hand). You might need to gently restrain the child's left hand to achieve the desired midline crossing motion with the right hand. Encourage the child to then hand the beanbag to the other therapist who is seated on the right side of the barrel. Have the therapist offer the beanbag to the second child, who should reach across her midline (with her left hand) for the beanbag and pass it back to the first therapist. The first therapist then hands the beanbag back to the second child who should take the beanbag with her right hand (for midline crossing) and hand it to the second therapist.

Repeat the activity several times with each child to encourage midline crossing from the opposite side. The children who are waiting for a turn can answer questions listed under the Language Prompts.

Helpful Hint: If a barrel is not available, the children can be positioned in chairs, on large blocks, or on another piece of therapy equipment (e.g., therapy balls with support for higher-functioning children who can keep their balance).

Language Prompts:
- Who is sitting on the barrel?
- What color/shape is the beanbag?
- Who has the beanbag now?

71

Copyright © 2004 LinguiSystems, Inc.

Activity 3: Tongue Lift ━━━━━━━━━━━━━━━━━━━━━━━━━━━━━

Have the children transition to the floor with their heads and backs against the wall to achieve stabilization of the head and jaw. Demonstrate tongue elevation by attempting to reach your nose with your tongue. Then have the children try it. Remind the children to let their tongues do the work, not their heads or necks.

Verbal prompts might be helpful (e.g., "Pretend you have peanut butter on your nose. Lick it off with your tongue."). Head and jaw stabilization may need to be assisted with physical prompts (e.g., hold the child's head with your hands on her cheeks or hold the child's head with one hand on top of her head and one under her chin).

Variation: Have the children kneel at a table. As a prompt, have them place their chins on the table so their heads cannot easily move forward or backward.

Activity 4: Cookie Lick ━━━━━━━━━━━━━━━━━━━━━━━━━━━━━

Have the children remain seated on the floor with their heads and backs against the wall to achieve stabilization of the head and jaw. Show the children a sandwich cookie that has been separated into two halves. Use your tongue tip to lick off the cream of one half of the cookie. Make sure the children see how you use your tongue tip when you lick off the cream. Then lick off the cream of the other half of the cookie.

Then give one child at a time a cookie separated into halves. The child may be able to hold the cookie herself, but you may need to assist the child by holding the cookie in the right position. Encourage the child to lift her tongue to lick the cream off the cookie. After the child has attempted two licks on each cookie half, give her that half to eat as a reward. To ensure that the head and jaw remain stable, physical prompts may be necessary (e.g., hold the child's head with one hand on top of the child's head and the other under her chin). If you give the child a physical prompt, the other therapist may need to hold the cookie.

> (Note: The goal of this activity is tongue elevation, so it doesn't matter if the child gets any cream off the cookie when she licks it. Provide positive prompts, such as "I know this is hard, but you tried your best," or "Great try! I saw your tongue trying to lick the cream off," or "Sometimes I can't do it either.")

Language Prompts:
- How many cookies do I have?
- What color is the cookie?
- What is in the middle of the cookie?
- What are you doing with your tongue? *(licking the icing, lifting it)*
- What kind of cookies do you like?

Variation: Have the children lie on their stomachs in a prone position while licking the cookies.

Activity 5: Friendship Circle

Have the children sit close together in chairs or on the floor in a circle. Show them how to cross their arms and link hands with the children next to them on either side in a "Friendship Circle." Lead the children in a familiar, calming song such as "Twinkle, Twinkle Little Star" while they sway side to side, maintaining the crossed-hand link. After the song is completed, encourage them to give themselves "hugs" with their arms crossing midline and wrapping around their bodies.

Language Prompts:
- Who is sitting next to you?
- What are you doing with your hands/arms? *(holding hands, crossing arms)*
- While singing the song, have the children fill in missing words (e.g., "Twinkle, Twinkle, _____ star").
- Whose hands are you holding?

Wrap-Up: Reintroduce the bee puppet to end the group, say good-bye to the children, and direct them to the next classroom activity.

> Therapist: *"We're all finished! Let's say good-bye to Buzzy. Now it's time for (name of next classroom activity)."*

The classroom teacher then gives the children instructions about the next activity.

                    Copyright © 2004 LinguiSystems, Inc.

Week Three

Materials:
Buzzy Bee
rings cut from foam plates (use the same rings from October activities)
yardstick
pairs of mittens cut out of construction paper (one mitten per child, make all right mittens one color and all left mittens a different color)
masking tape
colorful seals (three per child and one per therapist, the seals should be the kind that require moisture to affix)
construction paper or thematic pictures for the children to put the seals on
jar of peanut butter
Ritz crackers (one per child and therapist)
plastic knife
paper plate

Greeting:
Have Buzzy Bee greet each child individually by saying, "Hi, (child's name)." Encourage each child to respond appropriately to the puppet with verbal or nonverbal language.

> *Therapist:*   *"It's time to say hello to Buzzy Bee! Hi, Kelci!"*
> *Verbal Child:*   *"Hi, Buzzy!"*
>
> *Therapist:*   *"It's time to say hello to Buzzy Bee! Hi, Maria!"*
> *Nonverbal Child:* *Child must initiate eye contact and wave or smile.*

Warm-Up Activity:
Have the children sit in chairs or on the floor. With the other therapist, demonstrate a two-person hand-clapping pattern. Hold your hands in front of your bodies with your palms facing each other. Touch hands. Crisscross your hands and have your palms meet again. Then uncross your hands and have your palms touch again. End the pattern with a clap. Model a four-word phrase such as "One, two, three, magic" as you touch, crisscross, uncross, and clap hands. Have each child do the pattern with each therapist, thereby getting two turns to practice the motions.

(Note: You might want the four-word phrase to reflect your classroom theme [e.g., "pink hearts, red hearts"].)

Variation: Have the children attempt the hand-clapping pattern with one another.

Copyright © 2004 LinguiSystems, Inc.

Activity 1: Robot Walk

Have the children sit in chairs. Demonstrate how to put on "robot arms" using the foam rings. Get in a high kneel position. Have the other therapist hand you a foam ring (requiring you to reach for it with an extended arm). Take the ring and slide it over your opposite hand and up your arm so it sits on your shoulder. Do the same thing on your other arm. Then place a ring on your head (the children love this!) to complete the robot "costume."

Knee walk (high kneel position) with your arms extended to reach the other therapist. As you knee walk, sing the following words to the tune of "Frère Jacques."

> I'm a robot. I'm a robot.
> Big and tall. Big and tall.
> Watch me be a robot. Watch me be a robot.
> I won't fall. I won't fall.

Have the other therapist hold the yardstick on the right end horizontally in front of you at chest level. Take one foam ring off your arm and slide it from left to right across the yardstick to achieve midline crossing across a horizontal plane. Either hand may be used to slide the ring across the yardstick. Do the same with the other rings you are wearing.

Then have each child do this activity. To keep the activity moving, several children can put on robot arms and knee walk across the room at the same time. All of the children can sing the robot song.

Language Prompts:
- What color are the rings?
- How many rings do you have?
- Where are the rings? (on my head, on my arms, on the yardstick)

Activity 2: Wall Walk

Have the children take turns taping their paper mittens horizontally in a straight line across the wall. The mittens should be placed at the children's eye level and should be taped on the wall in an alternating color sequence (e.g., red, blue, red, blue).

Then say, "Let's pretend our hands are feet and have them 'walk' along the wall." Place your hands on the first pair of mittens and demonstrate how to use your hands to "walk" along the wall as you touch each mitten with your hands, crossing midline with a hand-over-hand pattern. Have each child take a turn as you shadow behind them, verbally prompting them to use hand-over-hand as they touch the mittens (e.g., "Put this hand on the red mitten and put this hand on the blue mitten."). Physical prompts may also be used as needed (e.g., hold the child's hands and go through the motions with her). Generally the cues and prompts can be faded out after the first few.

Language Prompts:
- What color is your mitten?
- What color is (name of child)'s mitten?
- How many mittens are on the wall?
- Where are you going to put your hands? *(on the mittens, on the wall)*
- When/why do you wear mittens?

Activity 3: Tongue Lift

Have the children transition to the floor with their heads and backs against the wall to achieve stabilization of the head and jaw. Demonstrate tongue elevation by attempting to reach your nose with your tongue. Then have the children try it. Remind the children to let their tongues do the work, not their heads or necks.

Verbal prompts might be helpful (e.g., "Pretend you have peanut butter on your nose. Lick it off with your tongue."). Head and jaw stabilization may need to be assisted with physical prompts (e.g., hold the child's head with your hands on her cheeks or hold the child's head with one hand on top of her head and one under her chin).

Variation: Have the children kneel at a table. As a prompt, have them place their chins on the table so their heads cannot easily move forward or backward.

Activity 4: Seal Lick

Have the children remain on the floor. Show the children the seals and explain that the seals are like stickers, but you have to wet them to make them stick. Demonstrate how to use your tongue tip to lick one. Then give one seal to each child and have her lick the seal from bottom to top, using only her tongue. Head and jaw must be stable to achieve the desired tongue elevation.

Place the seals on paper that has a thematic picture drawn on it that relates to classroom or seasonal activities (e.g., snowmen seals on a winter scene) or on paper to create decorations. Give each child three seals to lick and place on the paper. You could also have the children place their seals on envelopes to simulate stamps (e.g., Valentine's Day project).

Language Prompts:
- What is on your seal?
- What should you do with the seal? *(lick it, put it on the paper)*
- Where did you put your seal? *(on the paper, on the snowman)*

Activity 5: Peanut Butter Lick

Warning: If peanut allergies are present, this activity cannot be used unless substitutions for peanut butter are made (e.g., cream cheese, butter, Cheese Whiz).

Have the children remain seated on the floor with their heads and backs against the wall to achieve stabilization of the head and jaw. Spread peanut butter on a Ritz cracker. Then demonstrate how to use your tongue tip to lick the peanut butter off of the cracker, which is held vertically in front of your mouth.

Then give each child a cracker with peanut butter on it. Hold the cracker for the child to lick. Encourage the child to use her tongue tip to achieve tongue elevation. After the child has attempted three tongue licks on the cracker, let her eat it. To ensure that the head and jaw remain stable, physical prompts may be necessary (e.g., hold the child's head with one hand on top of the child's head and the other under her chin). If you give the child a physical prompt, the other therapist may need to hold the cracker.

(Note: The goal of this activity is tongue elevation so it doesn't matter if the child gets any peanut butter off the cracker when she licks it. Provide positive prompts, such as "I know this is hard, but you tried your best," or "Great try," or "Sometimes I can't do it either.")

Language Prompts:
- Where are the crackers? *(in the box, on the table)*
- Where is the peanut butter? *(in the jar, on crackers, on tongue)*
- What are you doing with your tongue? *(licking the cracker, lifting it)*
- What shape is the cracker?

Activity 6: Friendship Circle

Have the children sit close together in chairs or on the floor in a circle. Show them how to cross their arms and link hands with the children next to them on either side in a "Friendship Circle." Lead the children in a familiar, calming song such as "Twinkle, Twinkle Little Star" while they sway side to side, maintaining the crossed-hand link. After the song is completed, encourage them to give themselves "hugs" with their arms crossing midline and wrapping around their bodies.

Language Prompts:
- Who is sitting next to you?
- What are you doing with your hands/arms? *(holding hands, crossing arms)*
- While singing the song, have the children fill in missing words (e.g., "Twinkle, Twinkle, _____ star").
- Whose hands are you holding?

Copyright © 2004 LinguiSystems, Inc.

Wrap-Up: Reintroduce the bee puppet to end the group, say good-bye to the children, and direct them to the next classroom activity.

Therapist: *"We're all finished! Let's say good-bye to Buzzy.*
Now it's time for (name of next classroom activity)."

The classroom teacher then gives the children instructions about the next activity.

Week Four

Materials:
Buzzy Bee
two child-sized chairs
two gift wrap tubes
one beanbag
animal crackers (two per child and therapists)
two squeeze tubes of icing (The icing should be different flavors.)
paper plate or small plastic container (for the animal crackers)

Greeting:
Have Buzzy Bee greet each child individually by saying, "Hi, (child's name)." Encourage each child to respond appropriately to the puppet with verbal or nonverbal language.

Therapist:	*"It's time to say hello to Buzzy Bee! Hi, Kelci!"*
Verbal Child:	*"Hi, Buzzy!"*

Therapist:	*"It's time to say hello to Buzzy Bee! Hi, Maria!"*
Nonverbal Child:	*Child must initiate eye contact and wave or smile.*

Warm-Up Activity:
Have the children sit in chairs or on the floor. With the other therapist, demonstrate a two-person hand-clapping pattern. Hold your hands in front of your bodies with your palms facing each other. Touch hands. Crisscross your hands and have your palms meet again. Then uncross your hands and have your palms touch again. End the pattern with a clap. Model a four-word phrase such as "One, two, three, magic" as you touch, crisscross, uncross, and clap hands. Have each child do the pattern with each therapist, thereby getting two turns to practice the motions.

(Note: You might want the four-word phrase to reflect your classroom theme [e.g., "pink hearts, red hearts"].)

Variation: Have the children attempt the hand-clapping pattern with one another.

Copyright © 2004 LinguiSystems, Inc.

Week Four, *continued*

Activity 1: Paddle Your Boat

Have the children sit on the floor, against the wall. Place the chairs in front of the children in a row. The chairs should be one behind the other, facing either to the left or to the right. The children seated on the floor should see a side view of the chairs.

Show the children the gift wrap tubes. Explain that the tubes are the oars and the children will have a chance to pretend to row a boat. Have two children sit on the chairs.

Give each one a tube and help them hold it on the left sides of their bodies using both hands. Have the group sing "Row, Row, Row Your Boat" as the children on the chairs pretend to row using the tubes. Remember to have the children keep both hands on the tube to achieve midline crossing. Repeat the activity on the children's right sides. Then have the other children take their turns.

Language Prompts:
- Who is sitting on the chairs?
- What are they holding?
- What should they do with the tubes? *(row, hold them)*
- Who is sitting at the front/back of the boat?
- Where could you go on a boat?

Activity 2: Pass the Beanbag

The children sit cross-legged (i.e., legs like a pretzel) on the floor in a circle. Have them put their left hands behind their backs so they don't use them. Start passing the beanbag around the circle, always passing to the right to reinforce the left-to-right pattern. Help the children as they reach across their midline with their right hands to take the beanbag and give it to the next child. Physical prompts (e.g., gently guide the child's hand behind his back, gently hold the child's hand behind his back) or verbal reminders (e.g., "Put that hand behind your back, Hide that hand.") may be necessary to help the children keep one hand behind their backs. You may want to sing a song as you pass the beanbag.

Language prompts:
- What color is the beanbag?
- Who has the beanbag?
- Who is sitting next to you?
- Where is the beanbag?
- Where is your left hand? *(behind my back)*

Activity 3: Icing Lick

Have the children remain seated on the floor. Pair two children together and have them sit with their backs against one another and their legs stretched out in front of them. This will help provide the support they need to maintain head and neck stabilization.

Show the children the icing and the animal crackers. Choose a flavor and demonstrate how to squeeze the icing onto the back of a cracker. Then hold the cracker vertically in front of your mouth and lick the icing with your tongue tip from bottom to top, while maintaining a stable head and jaw.

Give each child a turn to choose a flavor, squeeze the icing onto a cracker, and lick it while you hold the cracker. Remind the children to only use their tongue tips to achieve tongue elevation. Once the child has attempted three tongue licks on the cracker, let her eat it. To ensure that the head and jaw remain stable, physical prompts may be necessary (e.g., hold the child's head with one hand on top of the child's head and the other under her chin). If you give the child a physical prompt, the other therapist may need to hold the cracker.

(Note: The goal of this activity is tongue elevation, so it doesn't matter if the child gets any icing off the cracker when she licks it. Provide positive prompts, such as "I know this is hard, but you tried your best," or "Great try," or "Sometimes I can't do it either.")

If you don't want to work on squeezing, prepare the crackers in advance. If you want to work on spreading, use a Popsicle stick or plastic knife and a container of icing.

Language prompts:
- What flavor/color of icing did you choose?
- What animal shape is your cracker?
- What flavor/color did (name of child) choose?
- Where are the crackers? *(in the box, on the table)*
- Where is the icing? *(on the cracker, on my tongue)*

Variation: To further promote midline crossing, place the crackers on the child's right or left side. Encourage the child to reach across her midline for a cracker. You might need to gently hold her other hand to keep her from using it.

Activity 4: Friendship Circle

Have the children sit close together in chairs or on the floor in a circle. Show them how to cross their arms and link hands with the children next to them on either side in a "Friendship Circle." Lead the children in a familiar, calming song such as "Twinkle, Twinkle Little Star" while they sway side to side, maintaining the crossed-hand link. After the song is completed, encourage them to give themselves "hugs" with their arms crossing midline and wrapping around their bodies.

Week Four, *continued*

Language Prompts:
- Who is sitting next to you?
- What are you doing with your hands/arms? *(holding hands, crossing arms)*
- While singing the song, have the children fill in missing words (e.g., "Twinkle, Twinkle, _____ star").
- Whose hands are you holding?

Wrap-Up: Reintroduce the bee puppet to end the group, say good-bye to the children, and direct them to the next classroom activity.

> *Therapist:*   *"We're all finished! Let's say good-bye to Buzzy.*
> *Now it's time for (name of next classroom activity)."*

The classroom teacher then gives the children instructions about the next activity.

Copyright © 2004 LinguiSystems, Inc.

Extra Activities

Use extra activities to reinforce February's themes and to lengthen the sessions if needed. Here are a few ideas to get you started.

Speech
Tongue Elevation

- Have the children lick small lollipops (e.g., DumDums).

- Make ice-cream cones and have the children lick the ice cream.

- Have the children lick Popsicles.

- Have the children lick peanut butter or icing off their upper lips. Remind them to move their tongues across their top lip, going from one side to the other.

OT
Bilateral Motor Skills and Midline Crossing

- Play ball games, particularly catching and throwing with large and small balls.

- Draw large rainbows from left to right using several colors of crayon or chalk.

- Play T-ball games using a plastic bat and ball.

- Play games that involve waving flags or fairy "wands" made of a ruler and a foil-covered star (e.g., wave flags to patriotic music, use fairy wand to pretend to change children into animals or storybook characters).

- Have the children do activities that require dressing and manipulating fasteners on clothing (e.g., play dress-up, dress/undress a doll, puzzles with fasteners on them).

Copyright © 2004 LinguiSystems, Inc.

MARCH

Themes: Sound Recognition, Discrimination, and Pronunciation of Early-Developing Initial Sounds

Grasp

Rationale

Speech: To learn the characteristics and placement of specific early-developing initial sounds and to be able to discriminate and produce those sounds. Target sounds include /p, b, t, d, m/, and /n/.

OT: The children have now worked on trunk stability as well as control and placement of the hand through wrist mobility superimposed on stabilization. Now the focus moves directly to hand use, beginning with grasp. This month emphasizes building up the arches in the hand which is necessary for opposition and encourages a strong and steady grasp.

Helpful Hints:

 Keep Buzzy Bee within arm's reach so you can quickly access it during activities as needed.

 If behavior or attention is a problem, you may want to divide the children into two separate groups (or two lines, depending on the activity) to achieve more control of the group.

Week One

Materials: Buzzy Bee
two different-colored moistened sponges, cut in half
two chairs
two small spray bottles
paper towels
paper of various types and textures (e.g., newspaper, tissue paper, construction paper)
basket or bucket
picture of a snowman
easel (or masking tape)
beach ball
permanent marker to write letters on beach ball

Greeting: Have Buzzy Bee greet each child individually by saying, "Hi, (child's name)." Encourage each child to respond appropriately to the puppet with verbal or nonverbal language.

> Therapist: "It's time to say hello to Buzzy Bee! Hi, Evan!"
> Verbal Child: "Hi, Buzzy!"

> Therapist: "It's time to say hello to Buzzy Bee! Hi, Jamal!"
> Nonverbal Child: Child must initiate eye contact and wave or smile.

Warm-Up Activity: Have the children sit in a circle on the floor or in their chairs. Sit in the circle with the children and have the other therapist sit opposite you. Show the children two half sponges (different colors) that have been slightly moistened with water. (The sponge is moistened only to make it easier to squeeze. Wring it out before giving it to the first child.) Demonstrate how to squeeze the sponge with one hand. Then pass the sponge to the child next to you. Have the child squeeze the sponge and pass it to the next child. Have the children continue squeezing and passing the sponge around the circle. When the first sponge reaches halfway around the circle, start the second sponge in the same direction. Say the word "Stop" at various points during the game. When you stop, have the children answer questions like the following.

Language prompts:
- Who has the (color) sponge?
- Who gave you the (color) sponge?
- Who will you pass your sponge to?
- What color is your sponge?

Copyright © 2004 LinguiSystems, Inc.

Activity 1: Chair Wash

Have the children sit down. Place two chairs in front of the group and put several sheets of paper towels on the floor. Introduce a small spray bottle filled with room temperature water. Explain that the chairs need to be cleaned. Demonstrate how to position your dominant hand on the sprayer handle and spray water onto the chair. Have the other therapist use a firm grasp to pick up a sheet of paper towel and wipe the chair in a circular motion. Then have the children work in pairs, taking turns spraying and wiping.

Activity 2: Snowball Squeeze and Throw

Have the children remain seated. Place the various types of paper on the floor or on a table in front of the children. Put the target on the opposite wall (snowman drawn on paper and placed on easel or taped to the wall) with the basket underneath.

Pick up one sheet of paper and say, "Let's make pretend snowballs out of paper." Crumple the paper into a ball and throw it into the basket. Then make another paper ball and throw it at the snowman target.

Give each child an opportunity to make paper balls to throw into the basket and to throw at the target. Remind the child to use a firm grasp when picking up a sheet of paper. Encourage him to squeeze the smallest paper ball he can. Some children may need physical prompts or assistance to crumple the paper.

> (Note: Encourage the child to use his dominant hand when throwing the paper ball. Some children may need to use both hands.)

Language Prompts:
- Where did you throw the snowball? *(in the basket, at the snowman)*
- Where did you hit the snowman? *(his head, his belly)*
- Is your snowball big or little?

Variations
1. Move the children closer to the target.
2. Use different textures/weights of paper (e.g., tissue paper, newspaper, construction paper).

Activity 3: Beach Ball Sound Game

Before doing this activity, write a few or several consonants and vowels on the beach ball with a permanent marker, depending on the children's abilities. Allow time for the marker to dry so the writing doesn't smear.

Have the children sit with their legs crossed like a pretzel in a circle on the floor. Sit opposite the other therapist. Hold the beach ball and look at the letters your thumbs are touching. Say one of the sounds. (If no letters are near your thumbs, pick one of the closest letters.)

Demonstrate how to pronounce the sound in isolation, providing verbal, visual, and tactile cues as needed (e.g., /b/ "Put your lips together and pop them, Feel the air exploding from your mouth, Feel the tickle [vibration] on your neck, Watch my lips").

After producing the sound, throw the beach ball underhand to the other therapist, stressing that the ball is thrown gently. Have the other therapist take her turn and then call a child's name and throw the beach ball underhand to him. Encourage the child to catch the ball and look to see where his thumbs are. Assist the child in reading a letter near one of his thumbs and making the corresponding sound. Then have the child call a classmate's name and throw the ball to him. Direct the game so each child has a turn. Make sure eye contact is achieved before allowing the ball to be thrown. Verbal prompts may be necessary to gain the child's attention (e.g., "Name of child—look at me").

(Note: You might need to position the child to catch the ball by extending the child's arms out in front of him and providing support to the child's trunk or arms.)

Each sound can correspond to a familiar label.

/s/—the snake sound	What does a snake sound like? *(sssss)*
/n/—the horse sound	Let's be a horse. What does a horse sound like? *(neigh)*
/m/—the "mmm good" sound	What do you say when something tastes good? *(mmmm)*
/d/—the hammer sound	What does a hammer sound like when you bang nails with it? *(ddddd)*
/p/—the popcorn sound	Let's be popcorn in a pot. What does popcorn sound like when it's popping? *(ppppp)*
/h/—the dog sound	What does a dog do when he's hot? He pants. *(hhhhh)*
/g/—the baby sound	Let's pretend to be babies. What sound does a baby make? *(goo-goo, gah-gah)*

Variation: Roll the ball instead of throwing underhand.

Wrap-Up: Reintroduce the bee puppet to end the group, say good-bye to the children, and direct them to the next classroom activity.

> *Therapist:* "We're all finished! Let's say good-bye to Buzzy. Now it's time for (name of next classroom activity)."

The classroom teacher then gives the children instructions about the next activity.

Week Two

Materials: Buzzy Bee
two different-colored moistened sponges, cut in half
carpet squares (one per child and therapist)
two clear plastic containers
two regular-sized sponges
paper towels
small table
sheet of paper with the letter P written on it
sheet of paper with the letter B written on it in a different color than P
flash cards (or objects) that begin with the initial /p/ sound* (page 143)
flash cards (or objects) that begin with the initial /b/ sound* (page 144)
box to hold the /p/ and /b/ flash cards (or objects)

*The number of flash cards will depend on how many children are in the group. You should have at least one for each child (e.g., If 12 children, have 6 for /p/ and 6 for /b/ or 12 for /p/ and 12 for /b/).

Greeting: Have Buzzy Bee greet each child individually by saying, "Hi, (child's name)." Encourage each child to respond appropriately to the puppet with verbal or nonverbal language.

> Therapist: "It's time to say hello to Buzzy Bee! Hi, Evan!"
> Verbal Child: "Hi, Buzzy!"

> Therapist: "It's time to say hello to Buzzy Bee! Hi, Jamal!"
> Nonverbal Child: Child must initiate eye contact and wave or smile.

Warm-Up Activity: Have the children sit in a circle on the floor or in their chairs. Sit in the circle with the children and have the other therapist sit opposite you. Show the children two half sponges (different colors) that have been slightly moistened with water. (The sponge is moistened only to make it easier to squeeze. Wring it out before giving it to the first child.) Demonstrate how to squeeze the sponge with one hand. Then pass the sponge to the child next to you. Have the child squeeze the sponge and pass it to the next child. Have the children continue squeezing and passing the sponge around the circle. When the first sponge reaches halfway around the circle, start the second sponge in the same direction. Say the word "Stop" at various points during the game. When you stop, have the children answer questions like the following.

Language prompts:
- Who has the (color) sponge?
- Who gave you the (color) sponge?
- Who will you pass your sponge to?
- What color is your sponge?

Activity 1: The Scratching Cat

Place a carpet square in front of each child. Pretend to be a cat and get down on all fours in a quadruped posture (e.g., on hands and knees in a standard crawling position). Take one hand and arch it, flexing all fingers. Use your flexed fingers to "scratch" the carpet like a cat would, moving your hand from the top of the carpet square to the bottom. As you do this, make a cat sound (meow). Repeat the motion a few times. Then have each child imitate it on his carpet square.

Activity 2: Bucket Fill

Place two clear plastic containers and a regular-sized sponge on a table. Fill one of the containers halfway with water. Explain that you need to move the water from one container to the other. Dip the sponge in the container with water and then move it above the second (empty) container. Use both hands to wring the sponge, making sure to squeeze tightly and twist it at the same time, allowing the water to fall into the empty container. Have the children take turns dipping and squeezing the sponges, watching as the water is transferred from one container to the other. Provide paper towels for the children to dry their hands on when their turns are finished.

Variation: Have the children use two sponges at a time.

Activity 3: /p/ and /b/ Box

Before this activity, put objects (or picture cards) that begin with /p/ and /b/ in a box.

Have the children sit in a horseshoe with their legs crossed like a pretzel with you at the open end of the horseshoe. Show the children the letters P and B written on separate sheets of paper. Name each letter and model its pronunciation. Provide verbal, visual, and tactile cues to help the children hear and see the difference between the sounds.

- /p/ is a soft (voiceless) sound and /b/ is a loud (voiced) sound.

- Put your lips together and make a pop sound for /p/ vs. a louder pop for /b/.

- Use your hand to simulate your mouth. Have your four fingers meet your thumb to imitate a closed mouth. As you say the /p/ or /b/, let your fingers fly open to simulate your mouth opening. Encourage the children to imitate this hand motion as they say the sounds.

- Feel the "tickle" (vibration) on your neck for /b/ vs. no "tickle" for /p/.

Put the papers with P and B on the floor in front of the children. Then show the children the box with the /p/ and /b/ objects. Have each child take turns putting his hand in the box and pulling out one item. Encourage the child to label the item while showing it to his peers. Have all of the children repeat the label. Then have the children guess which sound the item begins with. Model the word several times, placing emphasis on saying the word softly or loudly. Have the children repeat it each time. Then have the child put the object on either the P paper or the B paper.

Language Prompts:
- What did (name of child) pick?
- What is (name of child) holding?
- Where should (name of object) go? *(on the P paper or the B paper)*
- Did you pop your lips?
- Did your lips touch?
- Did you make a loud sound or a soft sound?
- Did you feel the tickle on your neck?

Wrap-Up: Reintroduce the bee puppet to end the group, say good-bye to the children, and direct them to the next classroom activity.

> *Therapist:* *"We're all finished! Let's say good-bye to Buzzy. Now it's time for (name of next classroom activity)."*

The classroom teacher then gives the children instructions about the next activity.

Materials: Buzzy Bee
two different-colored moistened sponges, cut in half
two small suitcases with rigid handles
two child-sized chairs
objects of various weights to place in the suitcases
small, smooth toys (e.g., balls, rubber animals, plastic beads)
sheet of paper with the letter T written on it
sheet of paper with the letter D written on it in a different color than P
flash cards (or objects) that begin with the initial /t/ sound* (page 145)
flash cards (or objects) that begin with the initial /d/ sound* (page 146)
play toolbox to hold the /t/ and /d/ flash cards (or objects)

*The number of flash cards will depend on how many children are in the group. You should have at least one for each child (e.g., If 12 children, have 6 for /t/ and 6 for /d/ or 12 for /t/ and 12 for /d/).

Greeting: Have Buzzy Bee greet each child individually by saying, "Hi, (child's name)." Encourage each child to respond appropriately to the puppet with verbal or nonverbal language.

> *Therapist:*   "It's time to say hello to Buzzy Bee! Hi, Evan!"
> *Verbal Child:*   "Hi, Buzzy!"
>
> *Therapist:*   "It's time to say hello to Buzzy Bee! Hi, Jamal!"
> *Nonverbal Child:* Child must initiate eye contact and wave or smile.

Warm-Up Activity: Have the children sit in a circle on the floor or in their chairs. Sit in the circle with the children and have the other therapist sit opposite you. Show the children two half sponges (different colors) that have been slightly moistened with water. (The sponge is moistened only to make it easier to squeeze. Wring it out before giving it to the first child.) Demonstrate how to squeeze the sponge with one hand. Then pass the sponge to the child next to you. Have the child squeeze the sponge and pass it to the next child. Have the children continue squeezing and passing the sponge around the circle. When the first sponge reaches halfway around the circle, start the second sponge in the same direction. Say the word "Stop" at various points during the game. When you stop, have the children answer questions like the following.

Language prompts:
- Who has the (color) sponge?
- Who gave you the (color) sponge?
- Who will you pass your sponge to?
- What color is your sponge?

Activity 1: Suitcase Carry

Before beginning the activity, place various objects in the suitcases to give them different weights. Place the suitcases several feet away from the child-sized chairs. Demonstrate how to grasp a suitcase with a firm hold and carry it to a chair. Lift the suitcase onto the chair, placing the suitcase on its side.

Give each child a turn to carry and lift a suitcase. Be sure to match the weight in the suitcase to a child who can handle it. This activity facilitates a strong grasp and then reinforces extension, trunk elongation, and trunk stability.

Activity 2: Hidden Treasure

Show the children a small, smooth toy of any type (e.g., ball, rubber animal). Explain that you are going to place the toy in your hand and fold your fingers over the toy so you can hold onto it tightly. Say to the other therapist, "Try to get the toy!" Then the other therapist should try to take the toy away from you by prying your hand open. As she pulls, demonstrate how to maintain a tight grasp on the toy so the other therapist must work to open your hand and get the toy.

Next give each child a toy to hold. Move around the circle of children and attempt to elicit a strong grasp from each of them as you try to pry their hand open and get the toy.

Then reverse the activity. Hide a toy in your hand. Have the children take turns trying to pry your hand open. This promotes finger flexion, palmar arching, and hand strengthening.

Activity 3: /t/ and /d/ Toolbox Game

Before this activity, put objects (or picture cards) that begin with /t/ and /d/ in a play toolbox. If you do not have access to a toolbox, use a long, rectangular plastic container with a flip-up lid.

Have the children sit with their legs crossed like a pretzel in a horseshoe with you at the open end of the horseshoe. Show the children the letters T and D written on separate sheets of paper. Name each letter and model its pronunciation. Provide verbal, visual, and tactile cues to help the children hear and see the difference between the sounds.

- /t/ is a soft (voiceless) sound and /d/ is a loud (voiced) sound.

- Feel the "tickle" (vibration) on your neck for /d/ vs. no "tickle" for /t/.

- Have the children put their tongue tips behind their top teeth.

- Use your hands to simulate your mouth. Place your hands in a "T" (time-out) position (i.e., right hand is vertical, left hand is horizontal on top of right hand). As you say the /t/ sound, make your right hand simulate the tongue tip making contact with the alveolar ridge. When you say the /d/ sound, have your right hand move up and touch your left hand with a little more force. Have the children imitate the hand motions as they say the sounds.

Put the papers with T and D on the floor in front of the children. Then show the children the toolbox with the /t/ and /d/ objects. Have the children take turns opening the box and pulling out one item. Encourage the child to name the item while showing it to his peers. Have all of the children repeat the name. Then have the children guess which sound the item begins with. Model the word several times, placing emphasis on saying the word softly or loudly. Have the children repeat it each time. Then have the child put the object on either the T paper or the D paper.

Language Prompts:
- What did (name of child) pick?
- What is (name of child) holding?
- Where should (name of object) go? *(on the T paper or the D paper)*
- Is your tongue behind your teeth?
- Did you make a loud sound or a soft sound?
- Did you feel the tickle on your neck?

Wrap-Up: Reintroduce the bee puppet to end the group, say good-bye to the children, and direct them to the next classroom activity.

> *Therapist:*   *"We're all finished! Let's say good-bye to Buzzy. Now it's time for (name of next classroom activity)."*

The classroom teacher then gives the children instructions about the next activity.

Materials: Buzzy Bee
two different-colored moistened sponges, cut in half
large, soft rope (for tug-of-war)
blanket
bag of oranges (cut in half, one orange per every two children)
strainer
transparent pitcher
two hand juicers
small paper cups
sheet of paper with the letter M written on it
sheet of paper with the letter N written on it in a different color than M
flash cards (or objects) that begin with the initial /m/ sound* (page 147)
flash cards (or objects) that begin with the initial /n/ sound* (page 148)
play mailbox to hold the /m/ and /n/ flash cards (or objects)
mirror

*The number of flash cards will depend on how many children are in the group. You should have at least one for each child (e.g., If 12 children, have 6 for /m/ and 6 for /n/ or 12 for /m/ and 12 for /n/).

Greeting: Have Buzzy Bee greet each child individually by saying, "Hi, (child's name)." Encourage each child to respond appropriately to the puppet with verbal or nonverbal language.

Therapist:	*"It's time to say hello to Buzzy Bee! Hi, Evan!"*
Verbal Child:	*"Hi, Buzzy!"*

Therapist:	*"It's time to say hello to Buzzy Bee! Hi, Jamal!"*
Nonverbal Child:	*Child must initiate eye contact and wave or smile.*

Warm-Up Activity: Have the children sit in a circle on the floor or in their chairs. Sit in the circle with the children and have the other therapist sit opposite you. Show the children two half sponges (different colors) that have been slightly moistened with water. (The sponge is moistened only to make it easier to squeeze. Wring it out before giving it to the first child.) Demonstrate how to squeeze the sponge with one hand. Then pass the sponge to the child next to you. Have the child squeeze the sponge and pass it to the next child. Have the children continue squeezing and passing the sponge around the circle. When the first sponge reaches halfway around the circle, start the second sponge in the same direction. Say the word "Stop" at various points during the game. When you stop, have the children answer questions like those on the following page.

Language prompts:
- Who has the (color) sponge?
- Who gave you the (color) sponge?
- Who will you pass your sponge to?
- What color is your sponge?

Activity 1: Tug-of-War

Show the children how to play "tug-of-war." Place a blanket on the floor to use as a dividing marker. With the other therapist, demonstrate how to grip the rope with both hands using a supinated suitcase (hook) grasp (palm up) and pull against each other on opposing sides without stepping on the blanket.

Then have the children participate in the tug-of-war two at a time. Careful physical prompts are necessary to ensure that the activity is controlled and calm. If the children are capable, demonstrate and encourage a hand-over-hand motion on the rope.

Activity 2: Making Orange Juice

Before this activity, cut all of the oranges but one in half. Place the oranges, the hand juicers, the pitcher, and the strainer on a table.

Have the children sit in chairs around the table. Explain that you are going to make orange juice. Pass the whole orange around the circle of children for them to feel, smell, and grasp.

Then demonstrate how to take half of an orange, turn it upside down, and squeeze and rotate it on the juicer. Show the children the juice at the bottom of the juicer. You can also squeeze the orange half directly into the juicer to extract extra juice as this further encourages hand strength and grasp.

Have the children take turns helping make the orange juice. Give a child an orange half and have him use the juicer. Then have him squeeze the orange half to get even more juice. When he is done, have him help pour his juice through the strainer into the pitcher.

After each child has had a turn, give each child a small sample of juice to taste.

Language Prompts:
- What is this? *(an orange)*
- What shape/color is the orange? *(round, orange)*
- Where is the juice? *(in the juicer, in the pitcher)*
- What are you doing with the orange? *(squeezing)*
- How does the juice taste?
- Does the juice smell good?

Week Four, continued

Activity 3: /m/ and /n/ Mailbox

Before this activity, put objects (or picture cards) that begin with /m/ and /n/ in a play mailbox. If you do not have access to a mailbox, you will need to make one from a shoebox. Make sure to tape the lid on so it doesn't fall off. Cut an opening in the box to simulate the door of a real mailbox.

Have the children sit with their legs crossed like a pretzel in a horseshoe with you at the open end of the horseshoe. Show the children the letters M and N written on separate sheets of paper. Name each letter and model its pronunciation. Provide verbal, visual, and tactile cues to help the children hear and see the difference between the sounds.

- Feel the "tickle" (vibration) on your nose for both sounds.

- Have the children put their lips together when producing /m/ and to put their tongue tip behind their top teeth for the production of /n/.

- Touch your lips with your index finger to remind the children about lip closure for /m/. You could also say, "Close your lips," or "Don't forget to make your lips touch."

- Use your hands to simulate your mouth. Place your hands in a modified "T" (time-out) position (i.e., right hand is vertical with fingers slightly bent, left hand is horizontal on top of right hand). As you say the /n/ sound, make the fingers on your right hand move up and gently touch your left hand to simulate the tongue tip making contact with the alveolar ridge. Have the children imitate this hand motion as they say /n/.

    (Note: It's important to have your fingers slightly bent so you can discriminate between /t/ and /d/ and now /n/. When you make the /n/ sound, you aren't using the tongue tip like for /t/ and /d/. Your tongue is slightly bent at the alveolar ridge.)

Put the papers with M and N on the floor in front of the children. Then show the children the mailbox with the /m/ and /n/ objects. Have the children take turns opening the box and pulling out one item. Encourage the child to name the item while showing it to his peers. Have all of the children repeat the name. Then have the children guess which sound the item begins with. Model the word several times, placing emphasis on saying the word with either lip closure or tongue elevation. Have the children repeat it each time. Then have the child put the object on either the M paper or the N paper.

Language Prompts:
- What did (name of child) pick?
- What is (name of child) holding?
- Where should (name of object) go? *(on the M paper or the N paper)*
- Was your tongue behind your teeth?
- Did your lips touch?
- Did you feel the tickle on your nose?

Helpful Hint: Have a mirror on hand so the children can watch themselves as they produce the words. The mirror will provide a visual prompt for children who need the extra help in determining whether they made lip closure or tongue elevation.

Wrap-Up: Reintroduce the bee puppet to end the group, say good-bye to the children, and direct them to the next classroom activity.

> *Therapist:*   *"We're all finished! Let's say good-bye to Buzzy. Now it's time for (name of next classroom activity)."*

The classroom teacher then gives the children instructions about the next activity.

97

Copyright © 2004 LinguiSystems, Inc.

Use extra activities to reinforce March's themes and to lengthen the sessions if needed. Here are a few ideas to get you started.

Speech	OT
Sound Recognition, Discrimination, and Pronunciation of Early-Developing Initial Sounds	**Grasp**

Speech

- Play the "Read My Back" game. Tape a flash card onto each child's back. Have the children sit in a circle facing clockwise (so they see the person's back). Have each child say the word taped to the child's back in front of him.

- Pull objects/flash cards out of a bag and label them.

- Roll a Ping-Pong ball over one flash card at a time and say what is on the card.

- Play "Pin the Tail on Flash Cards." Tape flash cards onto a wall. Give each child a tail. The child must place a tail on a flash card and say the target word. Depending on the child's skill level, a blindfold could be used.

- Put flash cards into envelopes. Give each child an envelope. Have the child open the envelope and name the picture. Then have each child pass his envelope to the child sitting next to him for additional practice.

OT

- Play putty or clay-squeezing games (e.g., make pretend water balloons and squeeze them, make pretend oranges and squeeze them).

- Use play sand or rice to promote hand cupping. Cup both hands like you are going to catch a ball and fill the "cup" with sand or rice.

- Use a hole puncher to punch holes into paper. Start with light paper (e.g., tissue paper).

- Squeeze glue from plastic glue bottles during art projects.

- Squeeze water or other liquids out of plastic squeeze bottles (e.g., ketchup or mustard bottles).

- Use a nasal suction bulb (i.e., the kind given out by hospitals when a baby is born) to make a feather or a cotton ball move on a flat, smooth surface. Nasal suction bulbs are also sold at drugstores. (If you don't have a nasal suction bulb, you can use a small turkey baster.)

APRIL

Themes: Sound Recognition, Discrimination, and Pronunciation of Later-Developing Initial Sounds

Finger Isolation and Pincer Grasp

Rationale

Speech: To learn the characteristics and placement of specific later-developing initial sounds and to be able to discriminate and produce those sounds. Target sounds include /k, g, f, v/, and /s/.

OT: The children need to be able to isolate and control their fingers individually to perform more precise fine motor tasks. A pincer grasp is basic to the manipulation of small objects for functional activities.

Helpful Hints:

 Keep Buzzy Bee within arm's reach so you can quickly access it during activities as needed.

 If behavior or attention is a problem, you may want to divide the children into two separate groups (or two lines, depending on the activity) to achieve more control of the group.

 Copyright © 2004 LinguiSystems, Inc.

Week One

(Note: For this month, the warm-up and the greeting are combined.)

Materials:
Buzzy Bee
two washable markers
smiley face stickers
farm animal figures
uncooked macaroni
toy frying pan or pot
toy fishing pole (wooden dowel, string, magnet)
Mouth Position cards (pages 168–172)
large paper clips

(Note: The fishing pole is for the third activity. To make the fishing pole, drill a hole at the top of a wooden dowel [approximately 26" long]. Put a piece of string through the hole and tie it in a knot. Tie a magnet to the bottom of the string and let it hang to the floor.)

Greeting/ Warm-Up Activity:
Before the activity, draw a face on the fleshy side of your index fingers (fingertips) with the marker. If you don't want to draw with a marker, use smiley face stickers.

Make a fist with each hand and hold up your index fingers so they face the other therapist. Have the other therapist hold Buzzy and greet you by name. In response, wiggle (flex and extend) your index fingers to say "Hello" as you respond to the greeting, pretending they are finger puppets. Then both therapists should go around the circle of children, drawing a face on the fleshy side of each child's index fingers or placing a smiley face sticker on them. Greet each child with Buzzy. Encourage each child to respond by isolating and wiggling her index fingers.

Therapist:	*"It's time to say hello to Buzzy Bee! Hi, Kelci!"*
Verbal Child:	*"Hi, Buzzy!"*

Therapist:	*"It's time to say hello to Buzzy Bee! Hi, Maria!"*
Nonverbal Child:	*Child must initiate eye contact and wave or smile.*

Copyright © 2004 LinguiSystems, Inc.

Activity 1: Barnyard Jump

Have the children lie on the floor in a prone position (on their stomachs) with their upper bodies propped up on their elbows. Lie in the same position and demonstrate how to use your hands to form a "fence." (The fence is formed by extending your index fingers toward each other so your fingertips touch.) Have the other therapist make a toy animal jump over your fence.

Then help each child isolate her index fingers and form a "fence" so you can make animals jump over it.

Language Prompts:
- What animal is this?
- What does the (name of animal) say? *(moo, baa, etc.)*
- Did (name of the animal) jump over the fence?
- Who jumped over the fence?

Variations
1. To add number concepts, have the animals jump over 1, 2, or 3 fences in a series.
2. To add spatial concepts, have the animals jump over the fence and go under the fence.

Activity 2: Feed Buzzy

Have the children sit against a wall or in chairs. Explain that Buzzy loves to eat macaroni. Show the children a dish of uncooked macaroni noodles. Demonstrate how to pick up a single macaroni noodle and put it in a small (toy) frying pan or pot using a pincer grasp. Have the children take turns using a pincer grasp to pick up noodles and put them in the pan.

After all the children have had a chance to put the macaroni in the pot, have them take another turn to take the macaroni out of the pot using a pincer grasp to feed Buzzy.

Variations
1. Have the children come to the center of the room using a high kneel walk.
2. Depending on the level of oral motor readiness of the children, a Cheerio or jelly bean can be substituted for the macaroni. With this variation, the children are rewarded by eating the Cheerio or jelly bean.

Copyright © 2004 LinguiSystems, Inc.

Activity 3: Fishing for Sounds

Before the activity, copy and cut apart the mouth position cards on pages 168-172 and place a large paper clip on each one.

Discuss fishing pole safety. Remind the children that every child must remain seated while one child takes her turn. There is to be no swinging of the string or magnet and no pointing the fishing pole at anyone.

Have the children sit with their legs crossed like a pretzel in a horseshoe with you at the open end of the horseshoe. Show the children the mouth position cards and the fishing pole.

Place the mouth position cards upside down on the floor. Demonstrate how to hold the fishing pole while "fishing" for a mouth position card. Once you "catch" a card, take it off the magnet and show it to the children. Label the sound on the card and then demonstrate how to pronounce the sound in isolation, paying attention to any verbal, visual, and tactile cues needed (e.g., for /b/—"Put your lips together and hide your teeth, Put your hand in front of your mouth and feel the burst of air."). Have the children repeat the sound.

Then have the children take turns fishing, starting with the child sitting at one end of the horseshoe. When the child is finished with her turn, she should hand the fishing pole to the child sitting next to her and ask, "Do you want a turn?" That child must respond appropriately for her skill level (e.g., verbal or nonverbal response).

Have each child "catch" a mouth position card and label the sound on the card after a therapist's model. Then encourage the child to teach her peers how to pronounce the sound and to have them repeat it.

Language Prompts:
- Did you use your lips or tongue to make that sound?
- Was your mouth open or closed?
- Did you smile (lip retraction) when you made that sound?
- Was it a soft or loud sound?

Helpful Hint: To achieve more postural stability, have the children sit in chairs in a large circle.

Wrap-Up: Reintroduce the bee puppet to end the group, say good-bye to the children, and direct them to the next classroom activity.

> *Therapist:* "We're all finished! Let's say good-bye to Buzzy. Now it's time for (name of next classroom activity)."

The classroom teacher then gives the children instructions about the next activity.

Materials:
Buzzy Bee
two washable markers
smiley face stickers
three paper chocolate chip cookies (circles cut from manila folders with
    brown spots drawn on them)
sheet of paper with the letter K written on it
sheet of paper with the letter G written on it in a different color than K
flash cards (or objects) that begin with the initial /k/ sound* (page 149)
flash cards (or objects) that begin with the initial /g/ sound* (page 150)
plastic bowling pins and balls
tongue depressors
mirror

*The number of flash cards will depend on how many children are in the group. You should have at least one for each child (e.g., If 12 children, have 6 for /k/ and 6 for /g/ or 12 for /k/ and 12 for /g/).

Greeting/ Warm-Up Activity:

Before the activity, draw a face on the fleshy side of your index fingers (fingertips) with the marker. If you don't want to draw with a marker, use smiley face stickers.

Make a fist with each hand and hold up your index fingers so they face the other therapist. Have the other therapist hold Buzzy and greet you by name. In response, wiggle (flex and extend) your index fingers to say "Hello" as you respond to the greeting, pretending they are finger puppets. Then both therapists should go around the circle of children, drawing a face on the fleshy side of each child's index fingers or placing a smiley face sticker on them. Greet each child with Buzzy. Encourage each child to respond by isolating and wiggling her index fingers.

Therapist:	"It's time to say hello to Buzzy Bee! Hi, Kelci!"
Verbal Child:	"Hi, Buzzy!"

Therapist:	"It's time to say hello to Buzzy Bee! Hi, Maria!"
Nonverbal Child:	Child must initiate eye contact and wave or smile.

Activity 1: "Where Is Thumbkin?" Song

Lead the children in the "Where Is Thumbkin?" song, demonstrating and encouraging correct finger isolation as indicated in the song's words (e.g., "Where is Thumbkin, Pointer, Tall Man, Ring Man, and Pinkie"). Emphasis should be on isolating the thumb, index, and middle fingers. Physical prompts may be necessary for some children (e.g., touch the correct finger to know which finger to lift, hold the finger in place).

Activity 2: Cookie Monster Game

Have the children lie prone on the floor with their upper bodies propped up on their elbows. (You may need to model this position.)

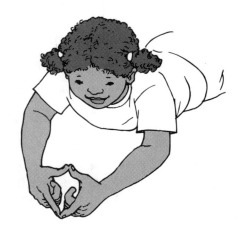

Show the cardboard cookies and explain to the children that they will all be "cookie monsters." Demonstrate how to isolate your thumbs and make your thumb tips touch each other. Then isolate and extend your index fingers, also making them touch. Rest the heel of each hand on the floor and have your fingers form a triangular opening or "mouth" to catch the cookies.

Have the other therapist drop one cookie into the opening. Use your index fingers and thumbs to pinch the cookie and trap it in the "mouth." Give each child several turns to catch cookies. For fun, encourage all of the children to make the /m/ sound when cookie is trapped.

(Note: You may want to make six cookies so two children can play at one time.)

Activity 3: /k/ and /g/ Bowling Pin Game

Have the children sit on the floor in a horizontal straight line facing you. Show the children the letters K and G written on separate sheets of paper. Name each letter and model its pronunciation. Provide verbal, visual, and tactile cues to help the children hear and see the difference between the sounds.

- Feel the "tickle" (vibration) on your neck for /g/ vs. no "tickle" for /k/.

- /k/ is a soft (voiceless) sound and /g/ is a loud (voiced) sound.

- Have the children put their tongue tips down behind their bottom teeth. Have the children do the mouth posture (open mouth, tongue tip down) and then produce the sound in isolation. Give each child a tongue depressor so they can hold their tongue tips down to form the correct placement for /k/ and /g/.

Put the papers with K and G on the floor in front of the children. Randomly place the /k/ and /g/ flash cards facedown on the floor. Put a bowling pin on top of each flash card. Demonstrate how to roll the ball to try to knock over a bowling pin. After you knock over a pin, turn the flash card over to see the picture. Say the word, placing emphasis on either the /k/ or /g/ sound. Provide cues as needed.

Then have the children take turns rolling the ball, knocking over a pin, and picking up a flash card. Encourage the child to name the picture while showing it to her peers. Have all of the children repeat the name. Then have the children guess which sound the item begins with. Model the word several times, placing emphasis on saying the word softly or loudly. Have the children repeat it each time. Then have the child put the object on either the K paper or the G paper.

Language Prompts:
- What picture is on your card?
- Does it start with a soft or a loud sound?
- Did you feel a tickle (vibration) on your neck?
- Was your mouth open or closed?

Helpful Hints: Use a mirror so the children can determine if they have their mouths in the correct position.

 If a child has difficulty obtaining the correct mouth posture for the production of /k/ or /g/, have the child lie on her back and open her mouth. (When you lie down and open your mouth, the correct mouth posture automatically occurs.) Have the child pronounce the /k/ or /g/ sound in isolation while in this position.

Wrap-Up: Reintroduce the bee puppet to end the group, say good-bye to the children, and direct them to the next classroom activity.

Therapist: *"We're all finished! Let's say good-bye to Buzzy. Now it's time for (name of next classroom activity)."*

The classroom teacher then gives the children instructions about the next activity.

Copyright © 2004 LinguiSystems, Inc.

Materials:
Buzzy Bee
two washable markers
smiley face stickers
teddy bear
several spring-type clothespins
stickers of items beginning with initial sounds previously targeted
   (e.g., /b/ ball, boat; /d/ dog, doll; /m/ mouse, map)
shoebox
a classroom theme-related outline of a picture (for the children to "color")
ink pad with washable ink
tray or table
large S's cut out of paper (one per child)
flash cards (or objects) that begin with /s/* (page 151-152)
Twister game (or different colored circles placed on the floor in your own
   design)
beanbag

*The number of flash cards will depend on how many children are in the group. You should have at least one for each child.

Greeting/ Warm-Up Activity:
Before the activity, draw a face on the fleshy side of your index fingers (fingertips) with the marker. If you don't want to draw with a marker, use smiley face stickers.

Make a fist with each hand and hold up your index fingers so they face the other therapist. Have the other therapist hold Buzzy and greet you by name. In response, wiggle (flex and extend) your index fingers to say "Hello" as you respond to the greeting, pretending they are finger puppets. Then both therapists should go around the circle of children, drawing a face on the fleshy side of each child's index fingers or placing a smiley face sticker on them. Greet each child with Buzzy. Encourage each child to respond by isolating and wiggling her index fingers.

Therapist: *"It's time to say hello to Buzzy Bee! Hi, Kelci!"*
Verbal Child: *"Hi, Buzzy!"*

Therapist: *"It's time to say hello to Buzzy Bee! Hi, Maria!"*
Nonverbal Child: *Child must initiate eye contact and wave or smile.*

Activity 1: Clothespin Pinch

Before the activity, put one sticker on each clothespin.

Show the children the clothespins, the teddy bear, and the shoebox. Explain that the bear is sad because all of his favorite things are missing from his box. The bear needs the children's help. To help the bear, the children must choose a clothespin and clip it onto the shoebox.

Have the other therapist show you three clothespins and ask you which special object you would like to give the bear. Name one of the stickers on a clothespin. Then open the clothespin by pinching it with your index finger, middle finger, and thumb. Place the clothespin on the edge of the shoebox.

Have the children take turns choosing a clothespin, naming the item on the sticker to reinforce production of the initial sound, and clipping the clothespin onto the shoebox. Only display three clothespins at a time. When a child chooses a clothespin, add another to always give a child three to choose from.

Language Prompts:
- Which toy are you giving the bear?
- What color is the toy?
- What should you do with the clothespin?
- Do you think the bear is happy now? Why?

Variations
1. Use wood or plastic clothespins of various sizes and levels of resistance.
2. Use chip bag clips for children with less strength and control.

Activity 2: Fingerprints

Show the children the paper with the outline picture on it. Place the paper on a tray. Explain to the children that they will "color in" the picture with their fingerprints.

Open the ink pad and demonstrate how to press your index finger onto the pad and then transfer the ink onto the construction paper. Repeat, using your thumb.

Then have each child take a turn, making several fingerprints.

(Note: You might want two or three different color ink pads to promote color concepts. You might also want to use scented ink pads to add sensory stimulation.)

Language Prompts:
- What color is this?
- Whose print is bigger?
- What are we coloring? (tree, flower, star, etc.)

Activity 3: /s/ Twister

Have the children sit on the floor in a horizontal straight line facing you. Show them a large letter S while you identify it and model how to pronounce it, emphasizing the fact that there is no tickle (vibration) on your neck when producing the sound. Instruct the children to put their teeth together and smile so they can achieve proper placement. (The prompt of using your hand and placing it in front of your mouth to feel the slight air stream coming from the front of the mouth will assist the children in producing the /s/ sound.)

Place a large S on the floor in front of each child and have them say the /s/ sound in isolation while tracing the letter S using their index fingers.

Put the Twister mat on the floor in front of the children. Place one flash card facedown or an object on each colored circle on the mat. Have the other therapist kneel on the other side of the mat, two to three feet away from the mat. Throw the beanbag underhand to her. When she catches it, she should high kneel walk to the Twister game and gently throw the beanbag onto one of the circles. Pick up the flash card or object and name it for the other therapist, putting emphasis on the /s/ sound.

Then have the children take turns catching the beanbag, knee walking to the Twister mat, and throwing the beanbag onto a circle. Give the child the flash card (object) on the circle. Encourage the child to name it while showing it to her peers. Model the word several times, emphasizing the /s/ sound.

After all of the children have repeated the word a few times, give the beanbag back to the child who tossed it. Have that child call the next child's name and toss the beanbag to her underhand. Remind the child not to throw the beanbag until eye contact is established. Then have the child knee walk back to her seat. Give each child a chance to be the receiver and the initiator of the beanbag toss.

Helpful Hint: You should pick up the beanbag and flash card/object to avoid having the children walk on the mat. Too much movement on the mat could cause the flash cards/objects to be moved or knocked over and could slow down the game.

Language Prompts:
- Who has the beanbag?
- Where did your beanbag land? *(on the mat, off the mat, on a red circle)*
- Who are you going to toss the beanbag to?
- Did you feel the air?
- What letter are you tracing?
- Are your teeth together (lips retracted)?

Wrap-Up: Reintroduce the bee puppet to end the group, say good-bye to the children, and direct them to the next classroom activity.

Therapist: *"We're all finished! Let's say good-bye to Buzzy.
Now it's time for (name of next classroom activity)."*

The classroom teacher then gives the children instructions about the next activity.

                     Copyright © 2004 LinguiSystems, Inc.

Materials:
Buzzy Bee
two washable markers
smiley face stickers
foil
chewy treats (e.g., gummy candy, fruit snacks)
clay, play dough, or Theraputty
pennies (four per child minimum)
child's purse with clasp or large change purse with clasp
fishing pole (from Week One)
sheet of paper with the letter F written on it
sheet of paper with the letter V written on it in a different color than F
Sea Creatures (pages 163—167, one per child)
flash cards that begin with the initial /f/ sound* (page 153)
flash cards that begin with the initial /v/ sound* (page 154)
large paper clips
mirror

*The number of flash cards will depend on how many children are in the group. You should have at least one for each child (e.g., If 12 children, have 6 for /f/ and 6 for /v/ or 12 for /f/ and 12 for /v/).

Greeting/ Warm-Up Activity:
Before the activity, draw a face on the fleshy side of your index fingers (fingertips) with the marker. If you don't want to draw with a marker, use smiley face stickers.

Make a fist with each hand and hold up your index fingers so they face the other therapist. Have the other therapist hold Buzzy and greet you by name. In response, wiggle (flex and extend) your index fingers to say "Hello" as you respond to the greeting, pretending they are finger puppets. Then both therapists should go around the circle of children, drawing a face on the fleshy side of each child's index fingers or placing a smiley face sticker on them. Greet each child with Buzzy. Encourage each child to respond by isolating and wiggling her index fingers.

Therapist: "It's time to say hello to Buzzy Bee! Hi, Kelci!"
Verbal Child: "Hi, Buzzy!"

Therapist: "It's time to say hello to Buzzy Bee! Hi, Maria!"
Nonverbal Child: Child must initiate eye contact and wave or smile.

Activity 1: Hidden Treat

Before the activity, place a chewy treat in a piece of foil and twist the ends closed. Make at least two for each child.

Demonstrate how to grasp the twisted ends between your thumbs and index fingers, one side with each hand, and rotate your wrists while maintaining your grasp to unwrap the treat.

Give each child a treat to unwrap. The children can eat the treat after they open it. You may want to give each child several pieces to unwrap for additional practice.

Activity 2: Penny Pull

Warning: Watch the children carefully when doing this activity to make sure the children are not putting the pennies into their mouths.

Before the activity, insert pennies into two small mounds of clay, play dough, or Theraputty. Place the pennies depending on the child's skill level (e.g., standing upright, lying flat).

Demonstrate how to use a pincer grasp to pull a penny out of the clay and place it in the change purse.

Have the children take turns pulling three to four pennies, one at a time, out of the clay and placing them in the purse. They can then practice closing and opening the purse's clasp for additional pincer grasp practice.

At the end of a child's turn, have the child push the pennies back into the clay to ready it for the next child, thereby providing an additional manipulative opportunity.

Helpful Hint: If you think a child is at risk for putting a penny into his mouth, use a larger manipulative item (e.g., checkers, large beads).

Variations
1. Have the pennies stand upright, lie flat, or be half buried in the clay.
2. Alter the clay to provide different degrees of resistance.

Copyright © 2004 LinguiSystems, Inc.

Activity 3: /f/ and /v/ Deep Sea Fishing Game

Before the activity, copy and cut apart the sea creatures on pages 163–167. Color them if you like. Paper-clip one flash card to the back of each sea creature.

Review fishing pole safety with the children. Remind them that every child must remain seated while one child takes her turn. No swinging the string or magnet and no pointing the fishing pole at any one.

Have the children sit with their legs crossed like a pretzel in a horseshoe with you at the open end of the horseshoe. Show the children the letters F and V written on separate sheets of paper. Name each letter and model its pronunciation. Provide verbal, visual, and tactile cues to help the children hear and see the difference between the sounds.

- /f/ is a soft (voiceless) sound and /v/ is a loud (voiced) sound.

- Feel the "tickle" (vibration) on your neck for /v/ vs. no "tickle" for /f/.

- Have the children bite their bottom lips for the production of /f/ and /v/. Show the children how to feel the burst of air coming from their mouths as they produce the sounds. First have the children imitate the mouth position (bite lower lip) and then produce the sound in isolation.

Put the papers with F and V on the floor in front of the children. Also place the sea creatures on the floor in front of the children with the sea creature facing up (the flash cards should not be visible). Demonstrate how to "catch" a sea creature using the fishing pole. When you catch a sea creature, take the card and sea creature off the fishing pole and show it to the children. Model the word, placing emphasis on either the /f/ or /v/ sound. Have the children repeat the word several times.

Have the children take turns catching the sea creatures. When a child catches a sea creature, encourage her to name the flash card while showing it to her peers. Have the children guess which sound the word begins with. Model the word several times, placing emphasis on saying the word softly or loudly. Have the children repeat it each time. Then have the child put the flash card on either the F paper or the V paper.

Turns should begin with the child sitting at one end of the horseshoe and continue around the horseshoe to the other end. When the child is finished with her turn, she should hand the fishing pole to the child sitting next to her and ask, "Do you want a turn?" That child must respond appropriately for her skill level (e.g., verbal or nonverbal response).

Helpful Hints:

 Use a mirror so the children can determine if they have their mouths in the correct position.

 To achieve more postural stability, have the children sit in chairs in a large circle.

Language Prompts:
- What picture is on the card?
- Did you bite your lip?
- Did you make a soft or loud sound?
- Did you feel the air?

Wrap-Up: Reintroduce the bee puppet to end the group, say good-bye to the children, and direct them to the next classroom activity.

Therapist: *"We're all finished! Let's say good-bye to Buzzy. Now it's time for (name of next classroom activity)."*

The classroom teacher then gives the children instructions about the next activity.

Extra Activities

Use extra activities to reinforce April's themes and to lengthen the sessions if needed. Here are a few ideas to get you started.

Speech	OT
Sound Recognition, Discrimination, and Pronunciation of Later-Developing Initial Sounds	**Finger Isolation and Pincer Grasp**

Speech

Sound Recognition, Discrimination, and Pronunciation of Later-Developing Initial Sounds

- Play a guessing game. Give clues to a target picture and have the children try to guess what it is.

- Create a mystery box with a shoebox and an old key. Place flash cards or objects with the target sound in the box. Have the children use the key to "unlock" the box and pull out an object or flash card to practice.

- Play a chocolate kiss game. Place a chocolate kiss on top of a flash card. After the child produces the word, she gets to eat the kiss.

- Toss hoops around a stuffed animal. When the child says the target word correctly, she tosses a hoop around the stuffed animal. (A *Sonny the Seal* game works well too.)

- Hang socks on a "clothesline" (rope tied between two chairs) with clothespins and put one flash card in each sock. Have the children take turns removing a sock from the clothesline and saying the word on the flash card. (Note: This activity also reinforces the child's ability to use a pincer grasp.)

OT

Finger Isolation and Pincer Grasp

- Tear paper of various thicknesses to make collages or pictures.

- Play with Lite Brite, Legos, or other small building toys.

- Play games using a toy piano keyboard for finger isolation (e.g., pretend to play songs, take turns pushing down one key).

- String small items (e.g., beads, Cheerios).

- Play games with a push button or toy telephone (e.g., pretend to call a family member, pretend to order pizza).

- Play with a spray bottle (e.g., squirt your hands, feet, and/or the grass, squirt water into a bucket).

Copyright © 2004 LinguiSystems, Inc.

MAY

Themes: Sound Recognition, Discrimination, and Pronunciation
of Previously Targeted Sounds in the Final Position

Separation of the Two Sides of the Hand
In-hand Manipulation Skills

Rationale

Speech: To use the skills previously learned about the characteristics and placement of specific sounds and to be able to discriminate and produce those sounds in final position and to attempt carryover from initial position to final position of a word.

OT: To execute more complex functional tasks, the child must learn to stabilize with the ulnar (pinkie) side of the hand and use precision and control with the radial (thumb and pointer finger) side. This is important for such activities as zipping (holding the fabric steady with the ulnar side, manipulating the zipper with the radial side), shoe tying, and developing a mature dynamic tripod grasp on a writing tool. To have good in-hand manipulation skills, the children need to practice squirreling small objects in their hands and being able to move items from palm to fingertips and from fingertips to palm using intrinsic hand muscles.

Helpful Hints:

 Keep Buzzy Bee within arm's reach so you can quickly access it during activities as needed.

 If behavior or attention is a problem, you may want to divide the children into two separate groups (or two lines, depending on the activity) to achieve more control of the group.

Week One

Materials: Buzzy Bee
Froot Loops
two small plastic bowls
pipe cleaners (one per child and therapist)
masking tape
small paper plates
pencil (for labeling the plates)
plastic tray
Cool Whip (thawed)
wet paper towels
small table
plastic eggs (at least one per child)
basket large enough to hold the plastic eggs
small pieces of paper with Vowel + Consonant nonsense syllables
(page 133)

Greeting: Have Buzzy Bee greet each child individually by saying, "Hi, (child's name)." Encourage each child to respond appropriately to the puppet with verbal or nonverbal language.

> *Therapist:*   *"It's time to say hello to Buzzy Bee! Hi, Evan!"*
> *Verbal Child:*   *"Hi, Buzzy!"*

> *Therapist:*   *"It's time to say hello to Buzzy Bee! Hi, Jamal!"*
> *Nonverbal Child:* *Child must initiate eye contact and wave or smile.*

Warm-Up Activity: Have the children sit in a line against a wall or in a semicircle on the floor. Explain that they are going to play a game by pretending that their fingers are legs that can hop, jump, walk, and run.

Demonstrate how to isolate your index finger and hold your hand so the tip of your finger is on the floor. "Hop" your index finger in front of your body along the floor. Have the children imitate you. Then demonstrate how to use your index and middle fingers to "jump, walk," and "run." Some children may need physical assistance to isolate the correct fingers. Have the children imitate each movement, making sure their fingers are doing the work, not their hands/arms.

(Note: You might want to provide a masking tape line for the children to make their fingers "walk" on.)

Variations
1. Limit the number of movements to hopping and jumping.
2. Have the children imitate movements with their thumbs and index fingers rather than index and middle fingers. Or have the children imitate a pivoting pattern with their thumbs and index fingers crossing over each other. This works on defining the web space (fleshy pad of skin connecting the thumb and index finger) as well as improving finger skills (e.g., finger isolation, controlling individual movement of the fingers).

Language prompts:
- What are your fingers doing? *(hopping, walking, jumping, running)*
- Are your fingers moving fast or slow?

Activity 1: Froot Loop Bracelets

Before the activity, put some Froot Loops in two bowls. Place small pieces of masking tape on each tip of the pipe cleaners to prevent exposed sharp edges.

Have the children sit on the floor in a horseshoe shape. Show the children the bowls of Froot Loops and the pipe cleaners. Explain that they will be making bracelets with the Froot Loops. Pick up one Froot Loop and demonstrate how to hold it in a pincer grasp and place it on a pipe cleaner. Circulate around the group with the other therapist, each of you holding a single pipe cleaner and a bowl of Froot Loops. Let each child place one Froot Loop on your pipe cleaner.

Then tell the children that you will string another Froot Loop on one of the pipe cleaners. Hold one hand open and flat, palm up and put your other hand behind your back. (It helps to use a verbal prompt such as "Make your hand flat like a table.") Have the other therapist place one Froot Loop on your open palm. Maneuver the Froot Loop from your palm to your fingertips (index finger and thumb). Then place the Froot Loop on a pipe cleaner the other therapist is holding.

Let each child attempt this activity. Some children may need physical prompts to remember to use only one hand (e.g., gently holding one hand behind the child's back). If time permits, let children maneuver more than one Froot Loop for additional practice.

For the last part of this activity, give each child several Froot Loops and a pipe cleaner of his own. Let the children make their own bracelets by stringing all of the Froot Loops they have. For this part of the task, bilateral skills and simple pincer grasp are being reinforced.

Place the bracelets on paper plates with each child's name to be distributed at snack time. It would probably be distracting to have the children wear the bracelets for the rest of the activities.

Activity 2: Cool Whip Fun

Before this activity, put some Cool Whip on the tray and place Froot Loops in it.

Have the children remain seated on the floor. Show the tray to the students and explain that some Froot Loops fell into the tray of Cool Whip. Demonstrate how to pick up a Froot Loop using your thumb and index finger and then put it in a plastic container. Give each child a chance to retrieve some Froot Loops from the Cool Whip. You can give each child a clean Froot Loop to eat after his turn.

Then tell the children that they need to hide one Froot Loop in their hands. Show them how to pick up and "hide" a Froot Loop in the ulnar (pinkie) side of your hand. While maintaining a grasp on the hidden Froot Loop, show the children how to retrieve another one from the Cool Whip using the radial side of your hand (index finger and thumb). Have each child who is able attempt this. For some children in the group, it may be appropriate for them to simply retrieve a Froot Loop from the Cool Whip without the additional challenge of holding the second Froot Loop in the ulnar (pinkie) side of the hand (ulnar stabilization).

Have wet paper towels available for the children to wipe their hands on after the activity.

Variation: Use other small food items in the Cool Whip for the children to retrieve, such as Cheerios, gummy candy, and Teddy Grahams.

Activity 3: Crack the Egg

Before the activity, cut apart the Vowel + Consonant nonsense syllables on page 133 or write them on separate slips of paper. Place one slip of paper in each plastic egg. Put all of the eggs in a basket.

Have the children sit in a horseshoe with their legs crossed like a pretzel with you at the open end of the horseshoe. Place a small table near you and put the basket filled with plastic eggs on the table. Tell the children that they are going to play a game called "Crack the Egg."

The target in this exercise is to produce the consonant in the final position of a nonsense syllable after a prolonged vowel sound (e.g., "eeeeg, ayayayayayg"). You can have the children produce long or short vowels.

Have the other therapist demonstrate how to crawl to the table with her hands flat on the floor, thereby promoting extra practice for wrist extension and postural stability. When she reaches the table, have her assume a high kneel position and extend her arm to reach for an egg in the basket, thus promoting trunk elongation. Have her "crack" the egg and pull it apart to get the slip of paper to hand to you. Read the nonsense syllable and have the other therapist repeat it. Continue by asking the other therapist, "What did you crack?"   The other therapist should respond by saying "egg," paying attention to the production of the final /g/ sound.

Then have the children take turns crawling up to get an egg. When they get to the table, they should reach for an egg, "crack" it, pull it apart, and hand the slip of paper to you so you can model the nonsense syllable. Then they should teach their peers how to pronounce the nonsense syllable and have their peers repeat it a few times. Use any necessary verbal, visual, and tactile cues from the previous months to help the children produce the target sound correctly.

/f/   Use your index finger and point to your lower lip. Have each child touch his lower lip with his index finger so he knows where to bite down to make the sound correctly.
Did you bite down?
Can you feel the air with your hand?
Is this a soft (voiceless) sound or a loud (voiced) sound?
Do you feel the tickle (vibration) on your neck?

/g/   Have each child imitate your mouth position of open mouth with tongue tip down.
Was your mouth open when you made the sound?
Did you smile when you made the sound?
Is this a soft (voiceless) sound or a loud (voiced) sound?
Do you feel the tickle (vibration) on your neck?

Turns should begin with the child sitting at one end of the horseshoe and continue around the horseshoe to the other end. When the child is finished with his turn, he must crawl back to his place in the horseshoe.

(Note: If you do not have access to plastic eggs, just put the slips of paper in the basket. You could also put the slips of paper in small bathroom cups and place them on the table.)

Variation: Use various sizes of eggs to reinforce the concept of *big/little* or *large/small*.

Wrap-Up: Reintroduce the bee puppet to end the group, say good-bye to the children, and direct them to the next classroom activity.

Therapist: *"We're all finished! Let's say good-bye to Buzzy. Now it's time for (name of next classroom activity)."*

The classroom teacher then gives the children instructions about the next activity.

                 Copyright © 2004 LinguiSystems, Inc.

Materials:
Buzzy Bee
two baby dolls
cotton balls
small stretchy men figures (one per child and therapist)
pennies (one per child and therapist)
sheet of paper with the letter P written on it
sheet of paper with the letter B written on it in a different color than P
sheet of paper with the letter M written on it in a different color than P
   and B
flash cards (or objects) that end with the final /p/ sound* (page 155)
flash cards (or objects) that end with the final /b/ sound* (page 156)
flash cards (or objects) that end with the final /m/ sound* (page 157)
several dimes
container to hold the dimes

*The number of flash cards will depend on how many children are in the group. You should have at least one for each child (e.g., If 12 children, have 4 or /p/, 4 for /b/, and 4 for /m/ or have 12 for /p/, 12 for /b/, and 12 for /m/).

Greeting:
Have Buzzy Bee greet each child individually by saying, "Hi, (child's name)." Encourage each child to respond appropriately to the puppet with verbal or nonverbal language.

> *Therapist:*   *"It's time to say hello to Buzzy Bee! Hi, Evan!"*
> *Verbal Child:*   *"Hi, Buzzy!"*

> *Therapist:*   *"It's time to say hello to Buzzy Bee! Hi, Jamal!"*
> *Nonverbal Child:*   *Child must initiate eye contact and wave or smile.*

Warm-Up Activity:
Have the children sit in a line against a wall or in a semicircle on the floor. Explain that the children are going to play a game by pretending that their fingers are legs that can hop, jump, walk, and run.

Demonstrate how to isolate your index finger and hold your hand so the tip of your finger is on the floor. "Hop" your index finger in front of your body along the floor. Have the children imitate you. Then demonstrate how to use your index and middle fingers to "jump, walk," and "run." Some children may need physical assistance to isolate the correct fingers. Have the children imitate each movement, making sure their fingers are doing the work, not their hands/arms.

(Note: You might want to provide a masking tape line for the children to make their fingers "walk" on.)

Variations
1. Limit the number of movements to hopping and jumping.
2. Have the children imitate movements with their thumbs and index fingers rather than index and middle fingers. Or have the children imitate a pivoting pattern with their thumbs and index fingers crossing over each other. This works on defining the web space (fleshy pad of skin connecting the thumb and index finger) as well as improving finger skills (e.g., finger isolation, controlling individual movement of the fingers).

Language prompts:
*   What are your fingers doing? *(hopping, walking, jumping, running)*
*   Are your fingers moving fast or slow?

Activity 1: "Ten Little Indians" Song

Have the children remain seated on the floor. Demonstrate how to isolate each finger sequentially as you sing the "Ten Little Indians" song. Then lead the children in the song while encouraging them to isolate their fingers as the numbers 1-10 are sung in the song. Some children may need physical prompts to do the finger motions. An approximation of the finger motions is acceptable.

Activity 2: Cotton Ball Baby Bath

Show the children two plastic baby dolls and explain that the babies need a "bath." Explain that you need two cotton balls to wash and dry a baby doll. Pick up one cotton ball and shift it to your palm, using fingertip to palm transition skills (i.e., moving an object from fingertips to palm using the small muscles in your hand). Then pick up the second cotton ball by pinching it between your thumb and index/middle fingers (radial pinch). Use the second cotton ball to "wash" the doll. To "dry" the doll, put down the cotton ball pinched between your thumb and index/middle fingers and move the other cotton ball from the ulnar side of your hand to your thumb and index/middle fingers.

Then have two children at a time "wash" and "dry" the dolls. Some children may need you to gently hold their non-dominant hands away or down as they grasp the cotton balls. This will insure that both cotton balls are held in one hand and the desired separation of the two sides of the hand is achieved.

Language Prompts:
*   Which part of the doll are you washing? *(nose, arms, legs, etc.)*
*   What are you washing the doll with?
*   How many cotton balls do you have?
*   What color are your cotton balls?
*   Are the cotton balls hard or soft?

Copyright © 2004 LinguiSystems, Inc.

Week Two, *continued*

Activity 3: Stretchy Men Game

Warning: Watch the children carefully when doing this activity to make sure the children are not putting the pennies into their mouths.

Have the children remain seated. Show the children a stretchy man and make him stretch by grasping his arms with your thumb and index fingers on each hand and gently pulling. Then give each child a stretchy man. Have the children stretch his arms and then his legs.

Next explain that the stretchy man is "hiding" his money. "Hide" a penny in each of your hands in the ulnar side (pinkie). Then pull the stretchy man's arms with a pincer grasp (thumb/index fingers) while simultaneously holding the pennies.

Help the children as needed to hide the pennies in the ulnar sides of their hands while holding on to the arms of the stretchy man with a pincer grasp. Have them practice stretching the rubber man's limbs while holding onto the pennies.

(Note: If you do not have access to stretchy men, you can use hair scrunchies.)

Activity 4: Dime Toss

Warning: Watch the children carefully when doing this activity to make sure the children are not putting the dimes into their mouths.

Before the activity, place the dimes in a container.

Have the children sit in a horseshoe with their legs crossed like a pretzel with you at the open end of the horseshoe. Show the children the letters P, B, and M written on separate sheets of paper. Name each letter and model its pronunciation. Have the children first imitate the mouth postures for the sounds and then produce each sound in the final position of a nonsense syllable. All verbal, visual, and tactile cues from previous lessons can be used to help the children hear and see the differences between the sounds. For example:

/p/   Put your lips together and pop them open.
       Did you feel the burst of air in front of your mouth?
       Did you pop your lips?
       Did you feel a tickle on your lips?
       Was this a soft (voiceless) sound or a loud (voiced) sound?
       Did you feel the tickle on your neck?

Put the papers with P, B, and M on the floor in front of the children. Randomly place the flash cards or objects on the floor. (The flash cards should be facedown.) Have the other therapist pick up one dime from the container using her thumb and index fingers.

Then she should toss the dime with an underhand throw using a pincer grasp onto a flash card or try to hit an object. You should pick up the dime and turn over the flash card or show the children the object. Have the other therapist name the picture/object, putting emphasis on the final /p/, /b/, or /m/ sound.

Have the children take turns picking up dimes, putting them in their hands, and tossing them onto a flash card or hitting an object. Encourage each child to name the picture/item while showing it to his peers. Have all of the children repeat the name. Model the word several times, emphasizing the final /p/, /b/, or /m/ sound. Have the children guess which sound the item ends with as they repeat the word after you. Then have the child put the object on the P paper, the B paper, or the M paper.

After the word has been practiced, have the child pick up the dime out of your hand using his thumb and index finger and drop the dime back into the container. Turns should begin with the child sitting at one end of the horseshoe and continue around the horseshoe to the other end.

Variation: Throw a larger coin, such as a quarter.

Wrap-Up: Reintroduce the bee puppet to end the group, say good-bye to the children, and direct them to the next classroom activity.

> Therapist: *"We're all finished! Let's say good-bye to Buzzy. Now it's time for (name of next classroom activity)."*

The classroom teacher then gives the children instructions about the next activity.

Copyright © 2004 LinguiSystems, Inc.

Materials:
Buzzy Bee
plastic tray
shaving cream
wet paper towels
several finger puppets
two sheets of construction paper (to make "curtains")
16 16-ounce plastic cups
masking tape
three Ping-Pong balls
flash cards (or objects) that end with the final /k/ sound* (page 158)
flash cards (or objects) that end with the final /g/ sound* (page 159)
two plastic containers, one with the letter K on it, one with the letter
   G on it (for the flash cards)

*The number of flash cards will depend on how many children are in the group. You should have at least one for each child (e.g., If 12 children, have 6 for /k/ and 6 for /g/ or have 12 for /k/ and 12 for /g/).

Greeting:
Have Buzzy Bee greet each child individually by saying, "Hi, (child's name)." Encourage each child to respond appropriately to the puppet with verbal or nonverbal language.

Therapist:	*"It's time to say hello to Buzzy Bee! Hi, Evan!"*
Verbal Child:	*"Hi, Buzzy!"*

Therapist:	*"It's time to say hello to Buzzy Bee! Hi, Jamal!"*
Nonverbal Child:	*Child must initiate eye contact and wave or smile.*

Warm-Up Activity:
Have the children sit in a line against a wall or in a semicircle on the floor. Explain that the children are going to play a game by pretending that their fingers are legs that can hop, jump, walk, and run.

Demonstrate how to isolate your index finger and hold your hand so the tip of your finger is on the floor. "Hop" your index finger in front of your body along the floor. Have the children imitate you. Then demonstrate how to use your index and middle fingers to "jump, walk," and "run." Some children may need physical assistance to isolate the correct fingers. Have the children imitate each movement, making sure their fingers are doing the work, not their hands/arms.

(Note: You might want to provide a masking tape line for the children to make their fingers "walk" on.)

Variations
1. Limit the number of movements to hopping and jumping.
2. Have the children imitate movements with their thumbs and index fingers rather than index and middle fingers. Or have the children imitate a pivoting pattern with their thumbs and index fingers crossing over each other. This works on defining the web space (fleshy pad of skin connecting the thumb and index finger) as well as improving finger skills (e.g., finger isolation, controlling individual movement of the fingers).

Language prompts:
- What are your fingers doing? *(hopping, walking, jumping, running)*
- Are your fingers moving fast or slow?

Activity 1: Shaving Cream Letters

Show the children how to use their hands to form the letters O and L. First extend your fingers to show an open palm. Next flex your fingers to have the tip of your thumb touch the tip of your index finger to form the O. Your other fingers also need to be bent to form the O. Then change your hand to form an L by fully opening the (web) space between your thumb and index finger. Extend your thumb horizontally and all other fingers vertically. Have the children practice forming the letters and transitioning from one letter to the other.

Next show the children a cafeteria tray with a light coating of shaving cream on it. Demonstrate how to isolate your index finger and draw the letter L in the shaving cream. Then smear the shaving cream to create a clear writing surface. Draw the letter O in the shaving cream. Present the tray to each child to practice writing each letter in the shaving cream.

While the children are forming the letters, have them imitate the sound that corresponds to the letter. You can also provide words for the children that correspond with the letter they draw in the shaving cream (e.g., "O is for open. O is for orange. L is for lion. L is for *light.*").

Helpful Hint: Use the wet paper towels for faster cleanup.

Language Prompts:
- What letter did you make?
- What color is the shaving cream?
- Does the shaving cream smell good?
- What does the shaving cream feel like? *(smooth, sticky, foamy)*

May
Let's Get Ready

Copyright © 2004 LinguiSystems, Inc.

Activity 2: Finger Puppet Show with a Curtain

Tell the children you are going to have a puppet show with the finger puppets. Hold the sheet of construction paper at its top outer edges with the ulnar (pinkie) side of your hands to form the "curtain" while extending your index fingers up, each with a finger puppet on it.

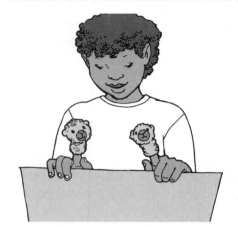

Then have two children at a time hold finger puppets and a curtain. They must maintain their grasp on the curtain while being able to manipulate their index fingers to make the puppets wiggle and move.

Activity 3: Cup Toss

Before you begin the activity, make the "Cup Toss" game. Tape one cup to another cup over the top edges so you have four in each row (four rows). It is also good to put tape around the perimeter of the cups to help keep the cups together. Then place a flash card or object in each cup. Place the K and G containers near the game on the floor.

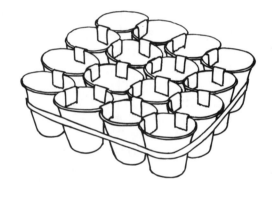

Introduce the letters K and G by modeling how to pronounce each one. Emphasize that there is no tickle (vibration) on your neck for the /k/ sound, but there is a tickle (vibration) on your neck for the /g/ sound. Remind the children to put their tongue tips down behind their bottom teeth when making /k/ or /g/. Have the children imitate the correct mouth position first (open mouth, tongue tip down) and then produce the sound in the final position of a nonsense syllable.

Have the children sit on the floor in two lines facing each other with the cups in between them. Get in a high kneel position near the cups and throw one Ping-Pong ball underhand into a cup. When the ball lands in one of the cups, knee walk over to the cup, reach down, take the ball out of the cup, and pick up the flash card or object. Name the flash card (or object), putting emphasis on the final /k/ or final /g/ sound.

Have the children take turns knee walking to the game, throwing the ball underhand, and getting a ball into a cup. When the ball lands in a cup, help the child retrieve the flash card (or object). Have the child name the flash card (object) while showing it to his peers. Have the children guess which sound the item ends with as they repeat the word after you. Model the word several times, placing emphasis on the final /k/ or /g/ sound. Have the children repeat it each time. Then have the child put the flash card (object) in either the container with the letter K on it or the container with the letter G on it.

Each child should be given two chances to sink the ball into the cup. If the child misses the cups on both attempts, have the child knee walk over to the cups and choose one flash card or object. Provide a lot of verbal praise (e.g., "You tried really hard, You threw the ball well, I like how you're kneeling.").

Language Prompts:
- Did you feel the tickle (vibration) on your neck?
- Did you make a soft (voiceless) sound or a loud (voiced) sound?
- Was your mouth open or closed?

Wrap-Up: Reintroduce the bee puppet to end the group, say good-bye to the children, and direct them to the next classroom activity.

> Therapist: *"We're all finished! Let's say good-bye to Buzzy.*
> *Now it's time for (name of next classroom activity)."*

The classroom teacher then gives the children instructions about the next activity.

Materials:
Buzzy Bee
bubble wrap
"candy" machine (plastic container with a lid, scissors, permanent marker)
pennies (three pennies per child and three per therapist)
treats (e.g., gummy candy, M&Ms)
flash cards with pictures that end with the final /s/ sound* (page 160)
flash cards with pictures that end with the final /t/ sound* (page 161)
flash cards with pictures that end with the final /d/ sound* (page 162)

(Note: The plastic container is used in the second activity. To make a candy "machine," cut a vertical slot in the lid big enough for a penny to slide through. Using a permanent marker, draw a rectangle around the slot to represent a vending machine. Glue pictures or stickers of candy on the container and lid.)

*The number of flash cards will depend on how many children are in the group. You should have at least one for each child (e.g., If 12 children, have 4 for /s/, 4 for /t/, and 4 for /d/ or have 12 for /s/, 12 for /t/, and 12 for /d/).

Greeting:
Have Buzzy Bee greet each child individually by saying, "Hi, (child's name)." Encourage each child to respond appropriately to the puppet with verbal or nonverbal language.

> *Therapist:* "It's time to say hello to Buzzy Bee! Hi, Evan!"
> *Verbal Child:* "Hi, Buzzy!"

> *Therapist:* "It's time to say hello to Buzzy Bee! Hi, Jamal!"
> *Nonverbal Child:* Child must initiate eye contact and wave or smile.

Warm-Up Activity:
Have the children sit in a line against a wall or in a semicircle on the floor. Explain that the children are going to play a game by pretending that their fingers are legs that can hop, jump, walk, and run.

Demonstrate how to isolate your index finger and hold your hand so the tip of your finger is on the floor. "Hop" your index finger in front of your body along the floor. Have the children imitate you. Then demonstrate how to use your index and middle fingers to "jump, walk," and "run." Some children may need physical assistance to isolate the correct fingers. Have the children imitate each movement, making sure their fingers are doing the work, not their hands/arms.

(Note: You might want to provide a masking tape line for the children to make their fingers "walk" on.)

Variations:
1. Limit the number of movements to hopping and jumping.
2. Have the children imitate movements with their thumbs and index fingers rather than index and middle fingers. Or, have the children imitate a pivoting pattern with their thumbs and index fingers crossing over each other. This works on defining the web space (fleshy pad of skin connecting the thumb and index finger) as well as improving finger skills (e.g., finger isolation, controlling individual movement of the fingers).

Language prompts:
*   What are your fingers doing? *(hopping, walking, jumping, running)*
*   Are your fingers moving fast or slow?

Activity 1: Bubble Wrap Pop

Have the children sit in a circle on the floor. Show the children how to pop a bubble on a sheet of bubble wrap by holding it vertically and using your thumb and index finger (on your dominant hand) to pop one.

Have the children take turns commando crawling (on their bellies) several feet across the room to you. Then help the child as needed pop two bubbles, making sure that he grasps the bubble correctly. Encourage the child to say the word "pop" as he pops each bubble. After the child pops the bubbles (or demonstrates an attempt to squeeze the bubble correctly), have him walk back to his seat.

Activity 2: Buzzy's Candy Machine

Warning: Watch the children carefully when doing this activity to make sure the children are not putting the pennies into their mouths.

Have the children remain seated on the floor. Place some pennies on the floor and show the children the plastic container. Have the other therapist walk to you using a high kneel position. When she reaches you, have her use her pincer fingers (thumb and index finger) to pick up one of the pennies. Hold the plastic container about six inches above her head and have her reach up to place the penny in the candy machine. (Note: Holding the container up requires arm extension and reach.) Have each child take a turn putting one penny into the candy machine.

Next explain that the candy machine needs more pennies to work. Repeat the high kneel walk over to the plastic container. This time, pick up two pennies using the same hand. To do this, pick up the first penny and shift it to your palm, using fingertip to palm translation skills (i.e., moving an object from fingertips to palm using the small muscles in your hand). Then pick up the second penny, holding in the radial (thumb/index finger) side of your hand. Put the second penny (already in your fingertips) into the candy machine first. Then move the palmed penny back to your fingertips and place it in the candy machine.

Have each child attempt this. They may need gentle physical prompts to remember to use only one hand to pick up and manipulate the pennies. Give each child a small treat or piece of candy (e.g., M&Ms) after he has put his pennies in the candy machine.

Variation: Use only one penny for the second part of the activity. Place one penny in the child's outstretched palm and encourage palm to fingertip translation of a single item (one penny) without stabilization (no second penny). Watch to make sure the child doesn't rest his hand against his chest to avoid true in-hand manipulation movements. Make sure that the child's other hand remains behind his back so all of the hand motions are done unilaterally.

Activity 3: Food for Buzzy

Before the activity, lean the flash cards against a wall with the pictures facing the wall. Have at least four flash cards for each sound (/s/, /t/, /d/).

Have the children remain seated on the floor with their legs crossed like a pretzel. Children should be seated in a horseshoe with you and the other therapist at the open end of the horseshoe. Tell the children that Buzzy is hungry and they need to feed him. Put Buzzy on your hand. Have the other therapist crawl on all fours with palms and fingers fully extended to the flash cards. When she reaches the flash cards, have her pick up one card using only her thumb and index finger to form a pincer grasp. Using wrist rotation, have her flip the flash card over to reveal the picture and name the item pictured on the card.

You should then model the word for the children, placing emphasis on either the final /s/, /t/, or /d/ sound. Have the children repeat the word several times and guess which sound the word ends with. After the other therapist pronounces the word, have her "feed" Buzzy by placing her flash card in his mouth.

Have the children take turns crawling to the flash cards, picking one up using the pincer grasp, flipping it over, and naming the picture. After the child practices the word, have him walk to Buzzy and "feed" him. When his turn is over, have him walk back to his seat.

Turns should begin with the child sitting at one end of the horseshoe and continue around the horseshoe to the other end. Depending on the child's skill level, the child can say the word only or say the word in a target phrase or sentence. For example, the child might say:

> I fe**d** Buzzy.
> Buzzy like**s** (name of picture).
> Ea**t** (name of picture).

Language Prompts:
- Did you feel the tickle on your neck? (for the production of /d/)
- Did you feel the air? (for the production of /s/ and /t/)
- Did you smile? (lip retraction)
- Was your mouth open?
- Did you make a soft (voiceless) sound or a loud (voiced) sound?
- Did you feel your tongue behind your teeth?

Wrap-Up: Reintroduce the bee puppet to end the group, say good-bye to the children, and direct them to the next classroom activity.

> *Therapist:*   "*We're all finished! Let's say good-bye to Buzzy. Now it's time for (name of next classroom activity).*"

The classroom teacher then gives the children instructions about the next activity.

Extra Activities

Use extra activities to reinforce May's themes and to lengthen the sessions if needed. Here are a few ideas to get you started.

Speech	OT
Sound Recognition, Discrimination, and Pronunciation of Previously Targeted Sounds in the Final Position	**Separation of the Two Sides of the Hand, In-hand Manipulation Skills**

Speech

- Play the "Hot/Cold" game. Hide flash cards or objects around the classroom and have the child look for them. Tell the child "hot" as he gets closer to an object or "cold" as he moves away from a flash card. When the child finds a flash card, have him name the picture on it.

- Toss wooden beads onto flash cards that are arranged on the floor or in the "Cup Toss" game. Pick up the bead, turn the card over, and have the child name the picture on the flash card. Encourage the child to teach the other children how to say the word pictured on the card.

- Hide flash cards or objects in a container filled with sand. Have the children take turns sifting through the sand to find the flash card or object. When the child finds one, have him name it.

- Throw beanbags onto paper lily pads. Place flash cards under the lily pads. When the child gets a beanbag onto a lily pad, have him identify the item on the flash card.

OT

- Practice in-hand manipulation skills by moving Cheerios, mini-marshmallows, or other small food items from fingertips to palm and back to fingertips.

- Have the children practice their scissors skills by cutting along lines of various lengths and directions (horizontal, vertical, diagonal). They can also cut out shapes, pictures from magazines, and/or coupons.

- Practice dressing dolls or play dress-up using clothes with buttons and zippers. You can also have the children practice fastening their own coats and jackets.

- Use markers and crayons for art activities. If the children are developmentally ready, use dot-to-dot or maze books. If the children are not developmentally ready, have them color on blank paper or in simple coloring books.

Copyright © 2004 LinguiSystems, Inc.

Vowel + Consonant Nonsense Syllables for Crack the Egg game
(Week One, Activity 3, pages 118–119)

These can be short or long vowels.

ab	eb	ib
ap	ep	ip
at	et	it
ad	ed	id
am	em	im
an	en	in
ak	ek	ik
ag	eg	ig
as	es	is
af	ef	if
av	ev	iv

ob	oob
op	oop
ot	oot
od	ood
om	oom
on	oon
ok	ook
og	oog
os	oos
of	oof
ov	oov

Copyright © 2004 LinguiSystems, Inc.

JUNE

Theme: Celebration of Skills

Rationale

Speech & OT: To encourage the children to use previously learned skills at an ice-cream party to celebrate the completion of the *Let's Get Ready* program and all of their hard work during the school year

Helpful Hints:

 Keep Buzzy Bee within arm's reach so you can quickly access it during the activity as needed.

 If behavior or attention is a problem, you may want to divide the children into two separate groups (or two lines) to achieve more control of the group.

(Note: Because school ends at different times in June, there is only one week of activities [making ice-cream sundaes]. If you wish to extend the program, refer to the Extra Activities at the end of each month and create your own lessons. Or repeat favorite activities. Make sure to include the Greeting, a Warm-Up activity, and the Wrap-Up.)

Week One

Materials: Buzzy Bee
vanilla and chocolate ice cream
two ice-cream scoops
plastic or Styrofoam bowls (one per child and therapist)
fudge and caramel syrup
M&Ms (at least four per child)
chocolate and rainbow sprinkles in plastic shaker containers
plastic spoons
two small trays with handles
napkins

Greeting: Have Buzzy Bee greet each child individually by saying, "Hi, (child's name)." Encourage each child to respond appropriately to the puppet with verbal or nonverbal language.

Therapist:	*"It's time to say hello to Buzzy Bee! Hi, Kelci!"*
Verbal Child:	*"Hi, Buzzy!"*

Therapist:	*"It's time to say hello to Buzzy Bee! Hi, Maria!"*
Nonverbal Child:	*Child must initiate eye contact and wave or smile.*

Before the activity, set up the tables with four different stations so the children can make their own ice-cream sundaes.

Station One: ice cream, ice-cream scoops, bowls

Station Two: fudge and caramel syrup

Station Three: M&Ms in a bowl

Station Four: chocolate and rainbow sprinkles, spoons, napkins, trays

Warm-Up Activity: Have the children sit on the floor in front of the tables with the ice-cream supplies. Sit on a chair in front of the children and explain to the children that they are going to have an ice-cream party to celebrate the end of the *Let's Get Ready* program and to celebrate the end of the school year.

Have the children play a "thumbs-up/thumbs-down" game in response to questions about eating ice cream and making sundaes. (You will be reinforcing supination and pronation of the forearm as you work on thumb isolation.) Example questions are on the next page.

Do you like ice cream? Yes! Put your thumbs up! (Rotate both wrists and isolate your thumbs, with your thumbs pointing up to the ceiling.)

Do you like bugs on your ice cream? No! Turn your thumbs down! (Rotate your wrists with thumbs still isolated and point them down to the floor.)

Do you like syrup on your ice cream? Yes! (rotate thumbs up)

Do you like syrup on your head? No! (rotate thumbs down)

Do you like candy on your ice cream? Yes! (rotate thumbs up)

Do you like candy on your feet? No! (rotate thumbs down)

Activity 1: Ice-Cream Fun

Have the children remain seated on the floor in front of the tables. Ask the children to raise their hands if they are ready for their ice cream (trunk elongation). Explain that the children will move to various stations to create their ice-cream sundaes. Point out the different stations.

Station One: Offer vanilla or chocolate ice cream. Have the child scoop some ice cream into a bowl (promotes wrist rotation and grasp).

Station Two: Offer fudge or caramel syrup (requires pronunciation of clear initial sounds). Have the child squeeze the syrup (from plastic squeeze type bottles) onto the ice cream (promotes hand strength and grasp).

Station Three: Offer M&Ms. Have the child name the colors she would like. Then have the child place three or four M&Ms on her sundae one at a time (requires pincer grasp).

Station Four: Offer chocolate or rainbow sprinkles. Have the child shake sprinkles onto her sundae (requires supination and pronation to invert the container and reinforces postural stability).

Have the children come up one at a time to make their sundaes. When a child is done at a station, the next child can move there. Have an adult in charge of each station.

When each child completes her sundae, have her carry the bowl to the table on the tray (uses bilateral skills and postural control). Carefully monitor this process to make sure the sundaes make it to the table.

The last, and best, part of this activity is eating the sundae! (Spoon use requires wrist rotation and management of a tool. Eating the ice cream elicits lip closure and tongue movements.)

Encourage the children to use language that promotes good manners and appropriate social skills, such as "Please" and "Thank you." Also encourage the children to talk and engage in verbal turn-taking with their peers while eating their ice cream.

Language Prompts:
- Would you like fudge or caramel syrup?
- Do you want sprinkles on your ice cream?
- What color are your sprinkles?
- Where is your ice cream? *(in a bowl)*
- What are you eating your sundae with? *(a spoon)*

Wrap-Up/ Good-Bye: Reintroduce the bee puppet to end the group and have him say good-bye to each child individually. Encourage each child to respond appropriately to Buzzy using verbal or nonverbal language skills.

Therapist: *"It's time to say good-bye to Buzzy Bee! Good-bye, Kelci!"*
Verbal Child: *"Good-bye, Buzzy!"*

Therapist: *"It's time to say good-bye to Buzzy Bee! Good-bye, Maria!"*
Nonverbal Child: *Child must initiate eye contact and wave or smile good-bye.*

Let the children hug Buzzy if they want to as they are saying good-bye. Then, ideally, the group will transition to an outdoor play session to expand the celebratory, end-of-the-year feeling.

Copyright © 2004 LinguiSystems, Inc.

JULY

Sunday	Monday	Tuesday	Wednesday	Thursday	Friday	Saturday
	Carry a 2-liter bottle across the kitchen to the table. (promotes postural control)	Take a deep breath and blow dandelions. (increases breath support)	Play games with a flashlight in your room at bedtime. (promotes midline crossing and visual motor skills)	Practice blowing bubbles. (increases breath support)	Clap your hands on soap bubbles to pop them as your parent blows them. (promotes bilateral hand skills and visual motor integration)	
	Hang from a monkey bar or swing on a swing. (promotes postural control, trunk elongation, and grasp)	Blow whistles outside. (increases breath support)	Use a paintbrush to paint with water on an outside wall or a fence. (encourages wrist extension and control)	Chew crunchy food items. (achieves jaw stabilization)	Have a barbecue. Chew small bites of a hamburger. (achieves jaw stabilization)	
	Carry a suitcase or old briefcase containing favorite toys around the house. (increases postural control and grasp)	Chew gummy food items. (achieves jaw stabilization)	Spray plants or flowers with a spray water bottle. (promotes grasp)	Hold crackers with your lips before eating them. (promotes lip closure)	Use sponges for outside cleanup jobs. Practice squeezing, wringing water out of sponges, and wiping. (promotes grasp and hand strength)	
	Practice wheelbarrel walks with an adult holding your legs. (promotes postural control and gives input to the palms of the hands)	Drink from a straw. (promotes lip closure)	Help rub sunscreen on both arms and legs. (provides tactile input and facilitates midline crossing)	Press your lips together and smile. Hold for 5 seconds. (promotes lip closure)	Lick an ice-cream cone. (promotes tongue elevation)	
	Cut out coupons from the Sunday newspaper with scissors. (promotes bilateral motor skills and grasp)	Try to touch your nose with your tongue five times. (promotes tongue elevation)	Play games with balls such as mini-golf, T-ball, or catch. (promotes midline crossing and bilateral motor skills)	Lick the cream off of a sandwich cookie. (promotes tongue elevation)	Roll like a log down a grassy hill. (promotes trunk elongation and provides movement input)	

Copyright © 2004 LinguiSystems, Inc.

AUGUST

Sunday	Monday	Tuesday	Wednesday	Thursday	Friday	Saturday
	Transfer play sand to a bucket using either your cupped hand (promotes palmar arches and cupping), your thumb and pointer fingers (promotes pincer grasp), or a spoon (promotes wrist motions).	Say these words: *bee, bay, beach, bike,* and *ball.* (promotes awareness of the /b/ sound and achieves lip closure)	Dress and undress a small fashion doll. (promotes finger strength and use of intrinsic hand muscles)	Find 5 objects that begin with the /p/ sound. Practice saying them. (promotes awareness of the /p/ sound and achieves lip closure)	Visit a zoo if you can. Make the specific sound of 5 different animals. (promotes awareness of mouth postures and discrimination of sounds)	
	Use a plastic knife to cut strawberries, bananas, and melon. Eat using a spoon or piercing with a fork. (promotes grasp and wrist control)	Wear red today. Find 3 other red items. (promotes color identification and recognition)	Put coins in a piggy bank. (promotes finger manipulative skills)	Help sort and match socks from the laundry. (promotes concept identification and recognition)	Practice folding napkins in half at meal time. (promotes wrist control and visual spatial skills)	
	Play with building toys with small pieces such as Legos. (promotes finger strength and flexion)	Practice these words: *wet, hot, boat, heat,* and *kite.* (promotes awareness of the /t/ sound and tongue elevation)	Practice dressing skills and the use of fasteners when changing clothes. (promotes functional bilateral hand skills)	Think of 10 food items that begin or end with /s/. Practice saying those words. (promotes awareness of the /s/ sound)	As you drive in the car, sing or recite your favorite nursery rhymes and songs. (promotes articulation skills)	
	Practice pouring water from one plastic container to another, using various sizes of openings and spouts. (promotes wrist control and postural stability)	Look for items that are *big* and *little.* (promotes concept recognition and identification)	Open small plastic jars with spices, peanut butter, or other foods. Unwrap a stick of butter or a chocolate bar. (promotes wrist rotation and finger manipulation skills)	Write on the sidewalk or driveway with chalk. Label the colors you use. (promotes color identification and recognition)	Brush your hair and teeth extra times. (promotes wrist control and supination/pronation of the forearm)	
	Play on a piano or computer keyboard. Try using fingers on both hands to press the keys. (promotes finger isolation and bilateral skills)	Find 10 items that begin with the initial /k/ sound. Say them. (promotes awareness of the /k/ sound)	Use dot-to-dot or maze books. Complete a page and color it in. (promotes pre-writing and finger strength skills)	Play Hopscotch. Put a word on each block to practice. Say the word as you jump on the square. (promotes articulation skills)	Read a storybook. Practice saying the names of pictures. Retell the story to your family. (promotes articulation and language skills)	

Data Tracking Sheet

Month _____ Week _____ Date _____

Therapy (circle)

Speech TX   Theme _____

Occupational TX   Theme _____

Activities

Names			

Key:

A	Absent
+	Performed task correctly
R	Refused to do task
NA	Needed assistance (Explain)
–	Can't perform task (Explain)

Copyright © 2004 LinguiSystems, Inc.

Example Data Tracking Sheet

Month **October**   Week **Week 1**   Date **10/12**

Therapy (circle)   **(Speech TX)**   Theme **breath support**

                   Occupational TX   Theme _____

Activities

Names	deep breath and blow	blow tissue	blow Ping-Pong ball
Abbey	+++++ completed 5 of 5	+++++ completed 5 of 5	+++++ completed 5 of 5
Brian	A	A	A
Chris	+++-- completed 3 of 5	--+++ completed 3 of 5	+++++ completed 5 of 5
Dana	----- couldn't protrude lips	NA Therapist squeezed cheeks	NA Therapist squeezed cheeks
Evan	R	R	R Threw balls
Francis	---++ completed 2 of 5	NA was eating tissues	NA also tried to eat balls

Key:		
A	Absent
+	Performed task correctly
R	Refused to do task
NA	Needed assistance (Explain)
–	Can't perform task (Explain)

          Copyright © 2004 LinguiSystems, Inc.

Example Data Tracking Sheet

Month __*October*__   Week __*Week 1*__   Date __*10/12*__

Therapy   Speech TX   Theme __*trunk elongation*__
(circle)
          (Occupational TX)   Theme _____

Activities

Names	extend arms over head	pop bubbles by clapping	
Abbey	+++++ completed 5 of 5	+++++ completed 5 of 5	
Brian	A	A	
Chris	R	NA couldn't open hand	
Dana	------ broken arm	------ broken arm	
Evan			
Francis	NA Therapist assisted	NA hand-over-hand	

Key:

A	Absent
+	Performed task correctly
R	Refused to do task
NA	Needed assistance (Explain)
–	Can't perform task (Explain)

Initial /p/

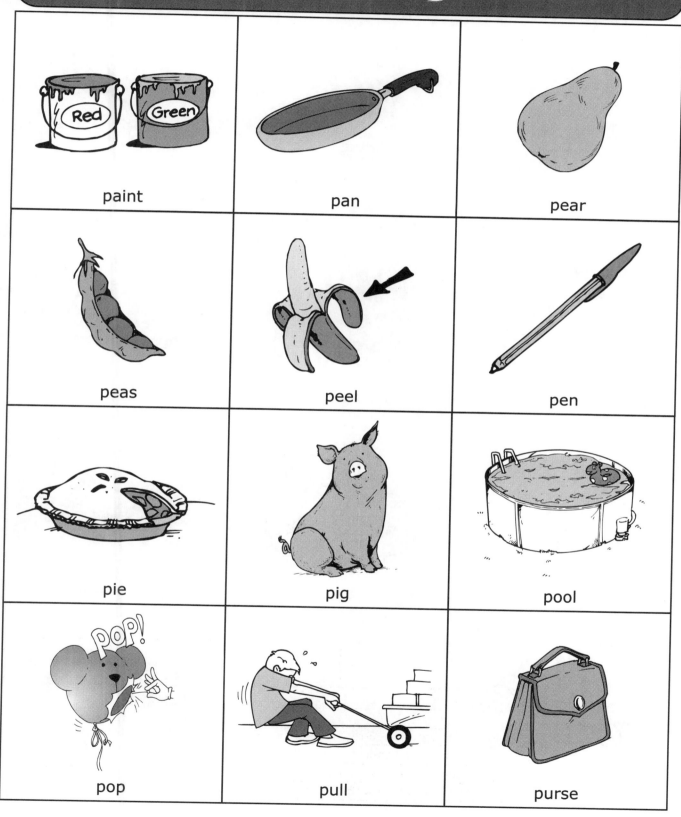

paint	pan	pear
peas	peel	pen
pie	pig	pool
pop	pull	purse

Initial /b/

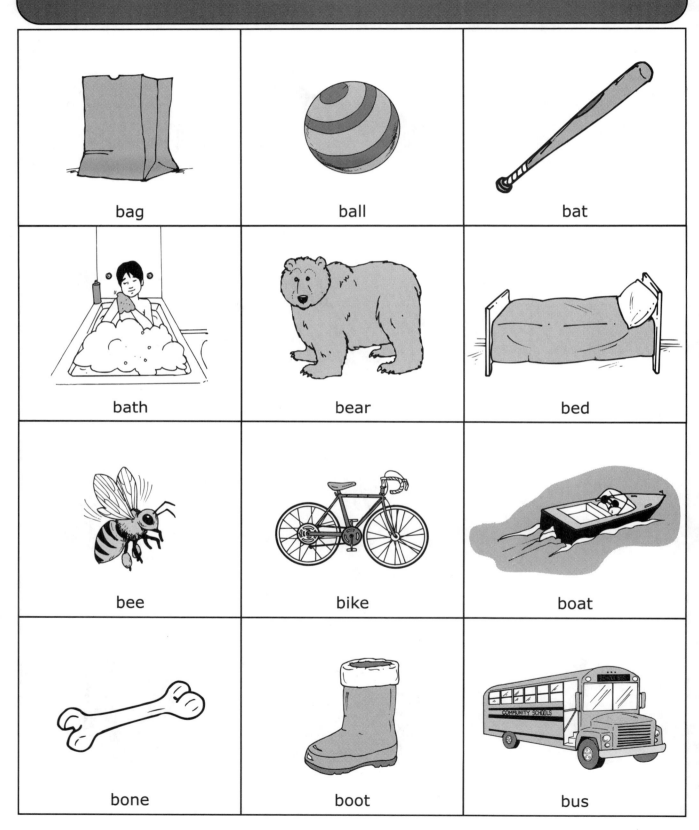

bag	ball	bat
bath	bear	bed
bee	bike	boat
bone	boot	bus

Initial /t/

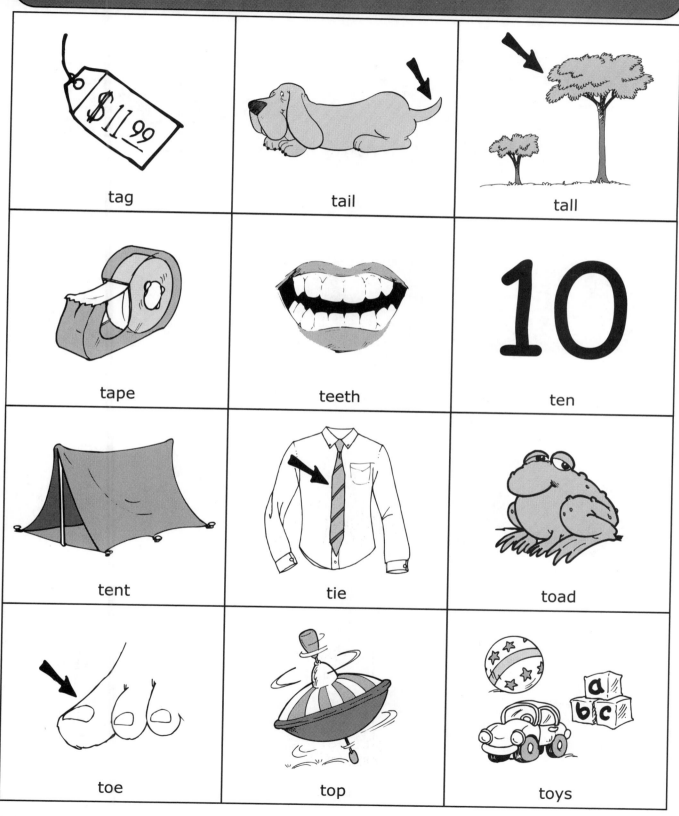

tag	tail	tall
tape	teeth	ten
tent	tie	toad
toe	top	toys

Initial /d/

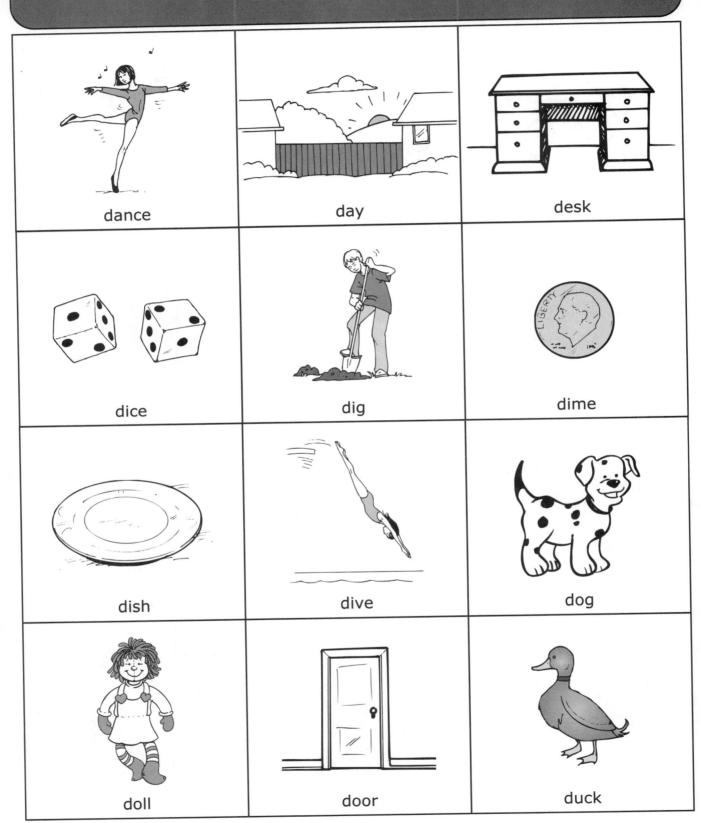

dance	day	desk
dice	dig	dime
dish	dive	dog
doll	door	duck

Initial /m/

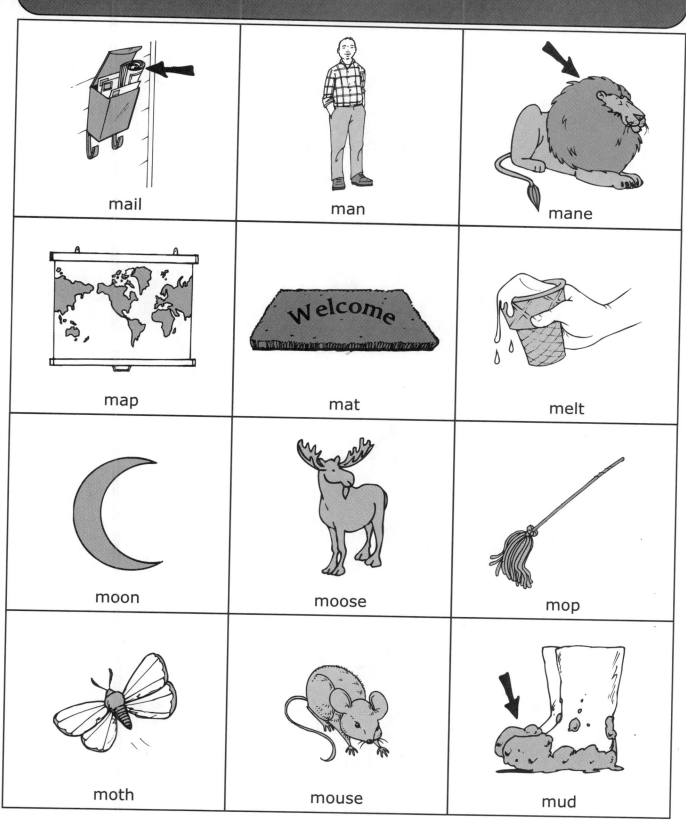

mail	man	mane
map	mat	melt
moon	moose	mop
moth	mouse	mud

Copyright © 2004 LinguiSystems, Inc.

Initial /n/

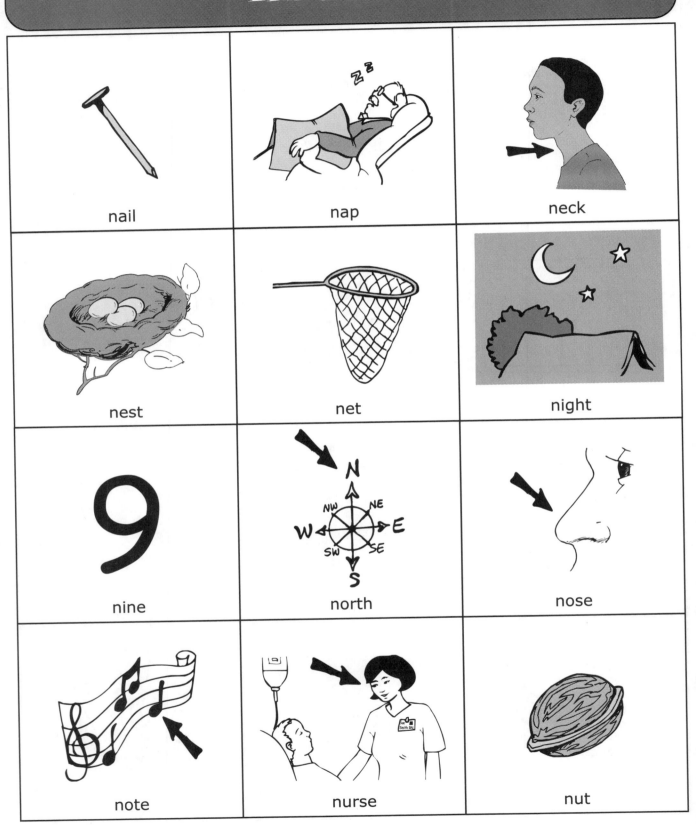

nail	nap	neck
nest	net	night
nine	north	nose
note	nurse	nut

Copyright © 2004 LinguiSystems, Inc.

Initial /k/

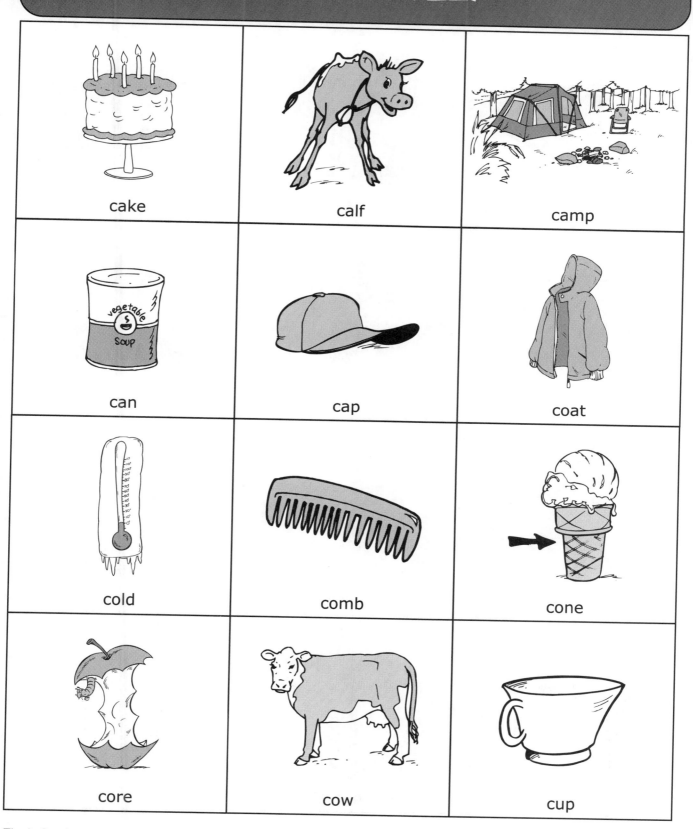

cake	calf	camp
can	cap	coat
cold	comb	cone
core	cow	cup

Initial /g/

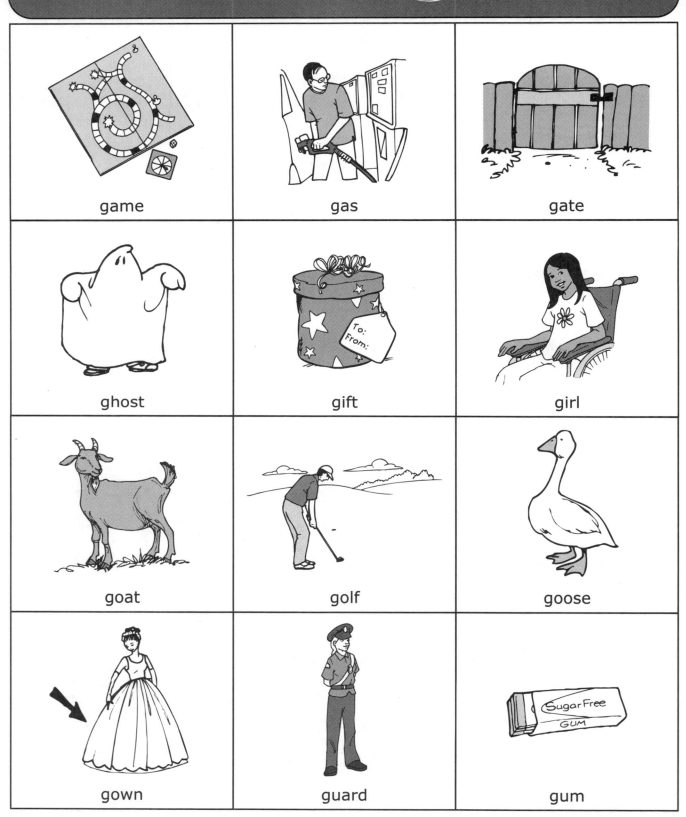

game	gas	gate
ghost	gift	girl
goat	golf	goose
gown	guard	gum

Initial /s/

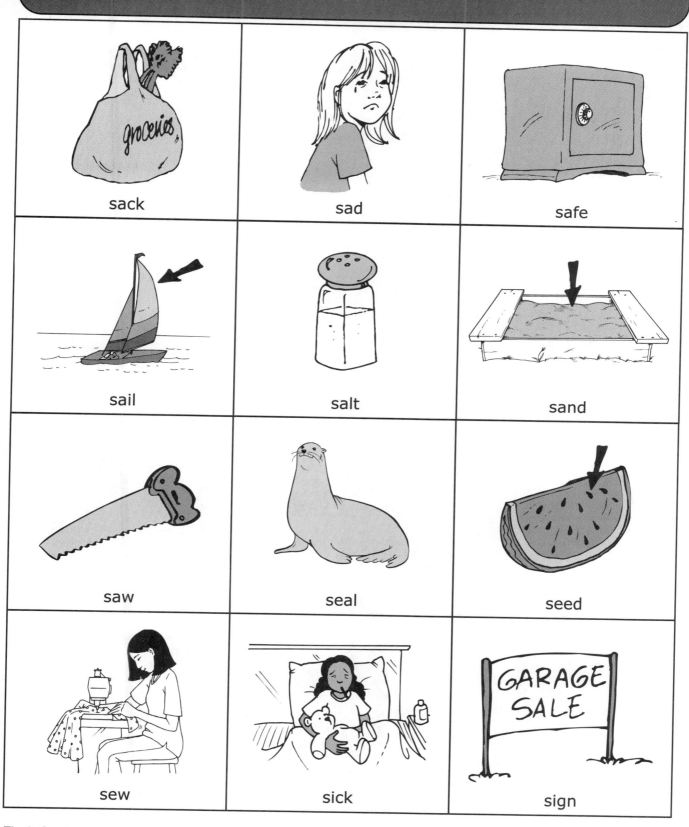

sack	sad	safe
sail	salt	sand
saw	seal	seed
sew	sick	sign

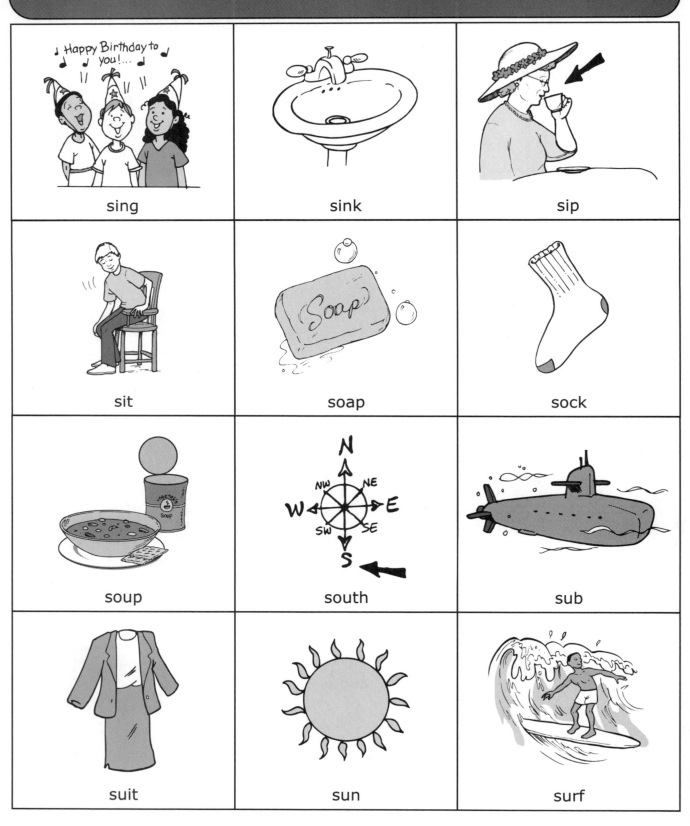

sing	sink	sip
sit	soap	sock
soup	south	sub
suit	sun	surf

152

Copyright © 2004 LinguiSystems, Inc.

Initial /f/

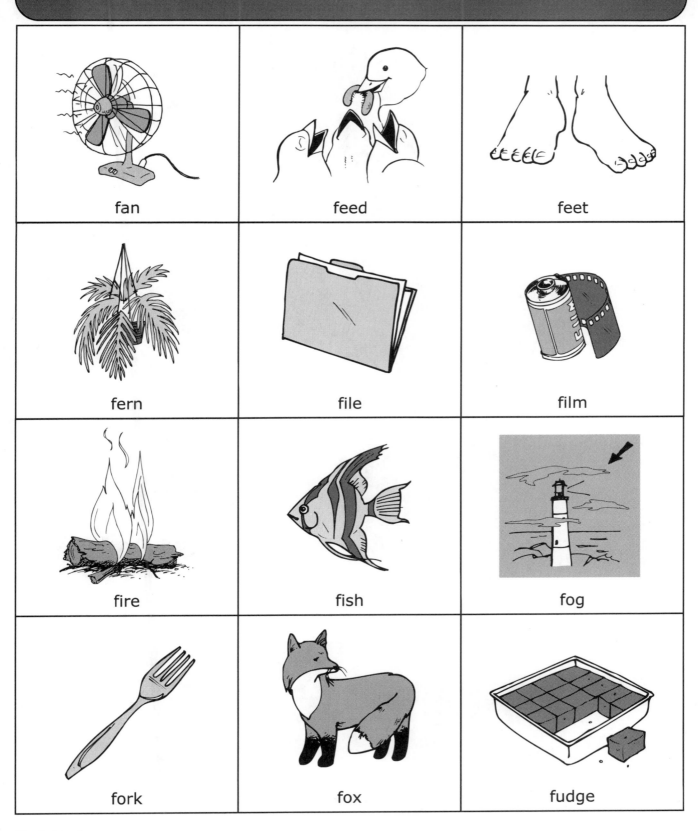

fan	feed	feet
fern	file	film
fire	fish	fog
fork	fox	fudge

Initial /v/

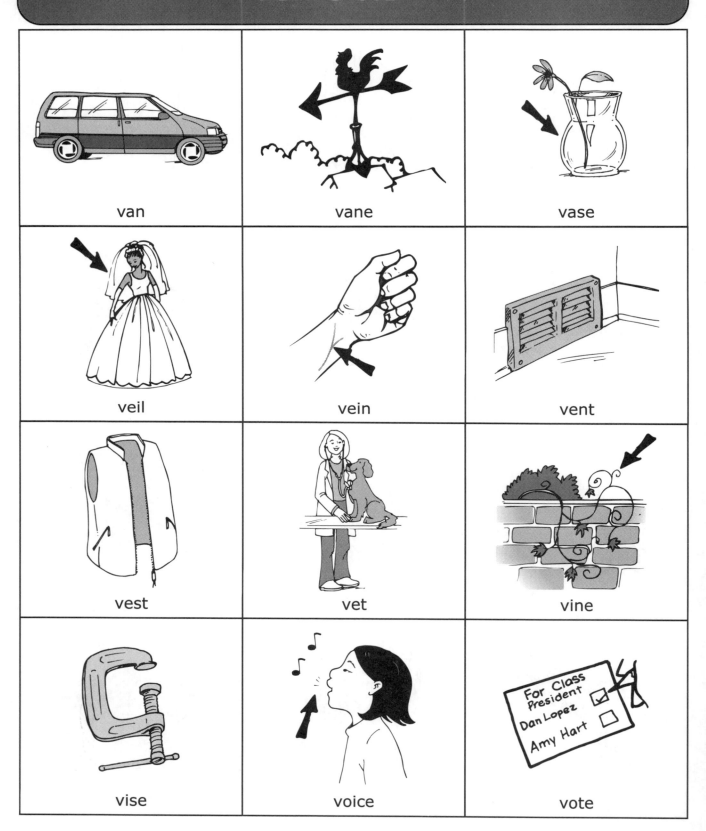

van	vane	vase
veil	vein	vent
vest	vet	vine
vise	voice	vote

Final /p/

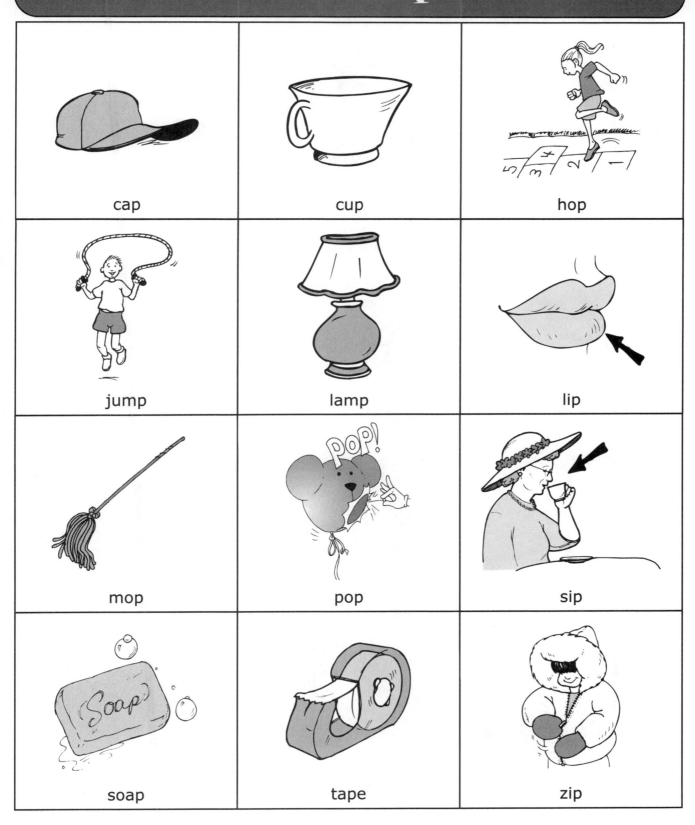

cap	cup	hop
jump	lamp	lip
mop	pop	sip
soap	tape	zip

Final /b/

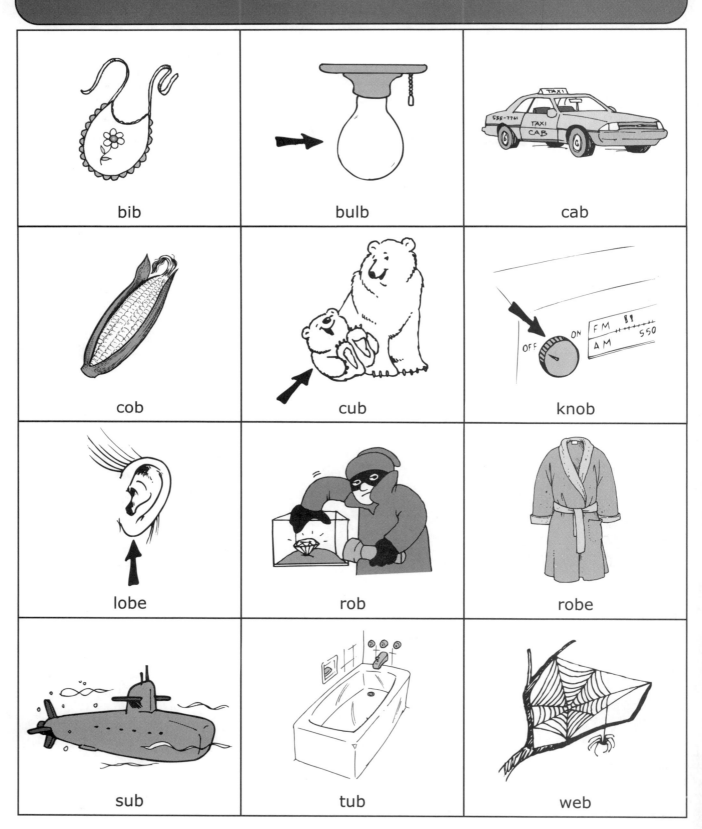

bib	bulb	cab
cob	cub	knob
lobe	rob	robe
sub	tub	web

Copyright © 2004 LinguiSystems, Inc.

Final /m/

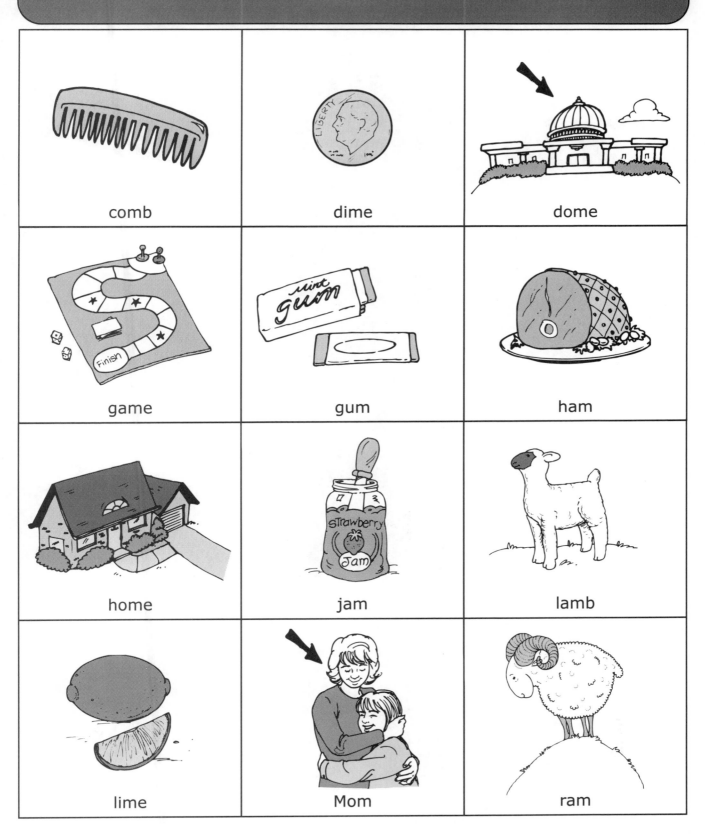

comb	dime	dome
game	gum	ham
home	jam	lamb
lime	Mom	ram

Final /k/

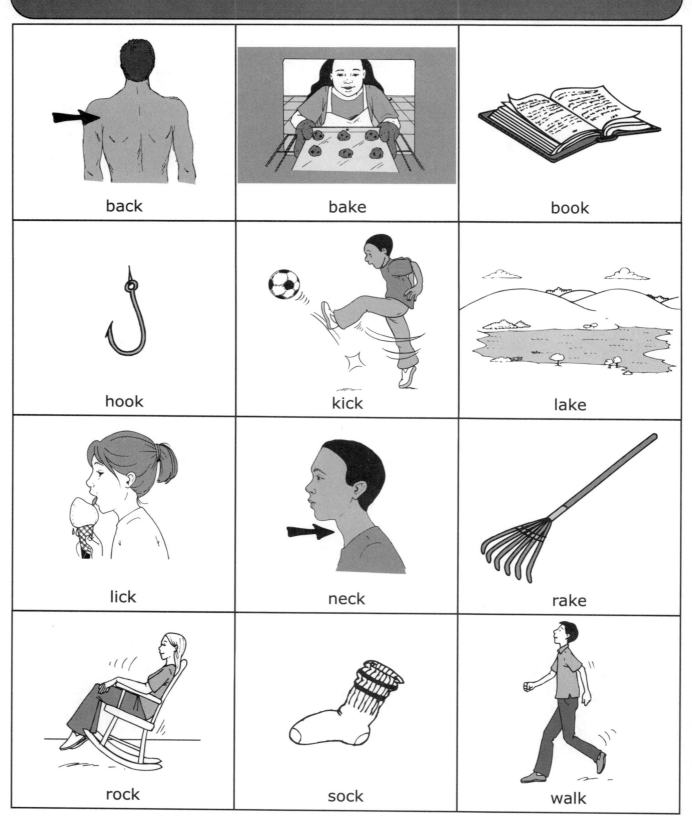

back	bake	book
hook	kick	lake
lick	neck	rake
rock	sock	walk

Final /g/

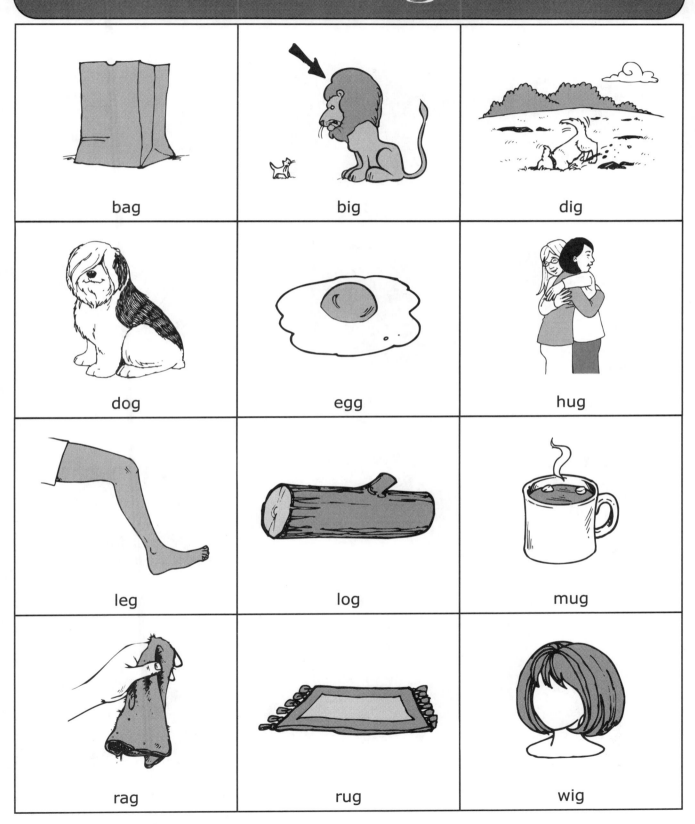

bag	big	dig
dog	egg	hug
leg	log	mug
rag	rug	wig

Copyright © 2004 LinguiSystems, Inc.

Final /s/

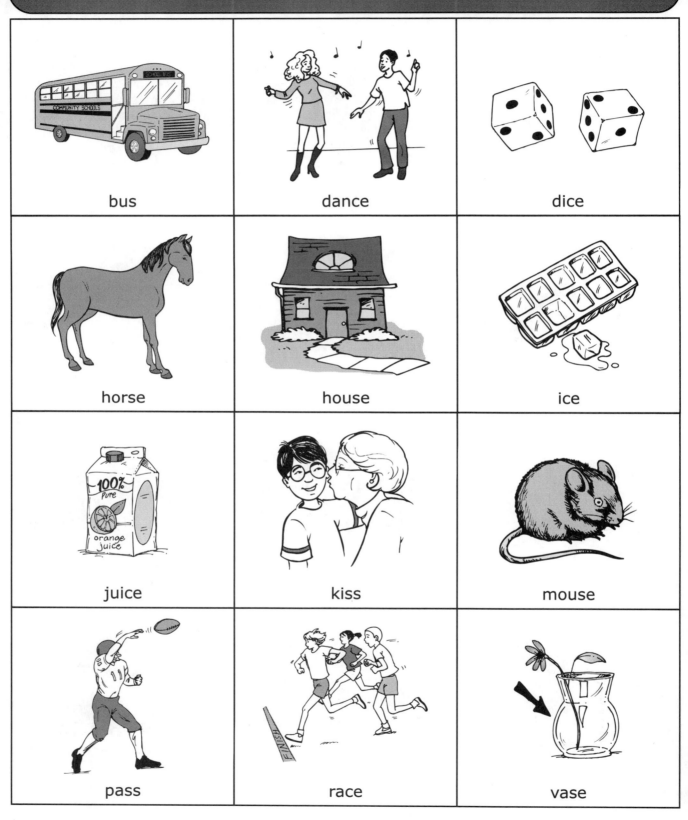

bus	dance	dice
horse	house	ice
juice	kiss	mouse
pass	race	vase

Final /t/

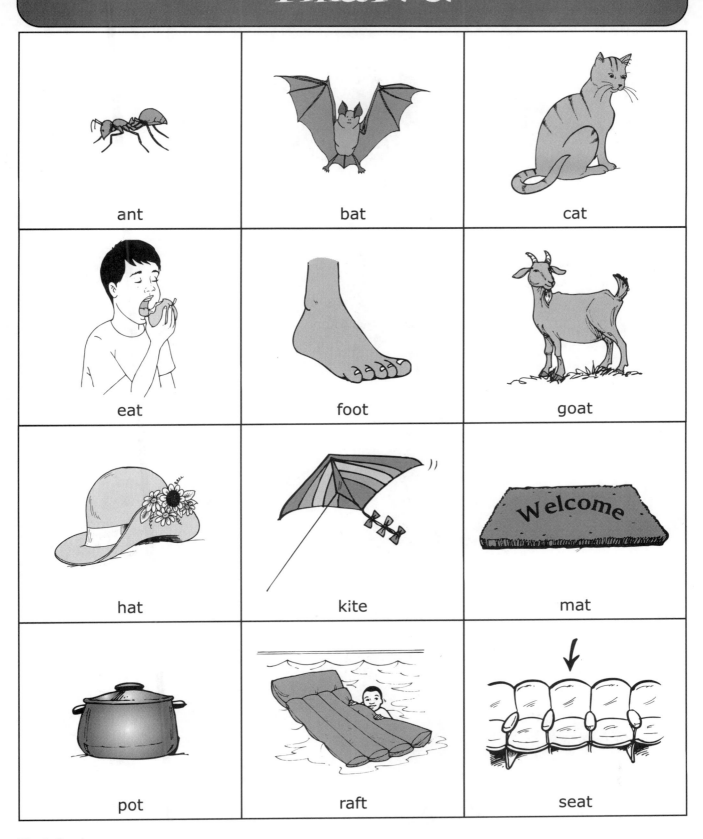

ant	bat	cat
eat	foot	goat
hat	kite	mat
pot	raft	seat

Final /d/

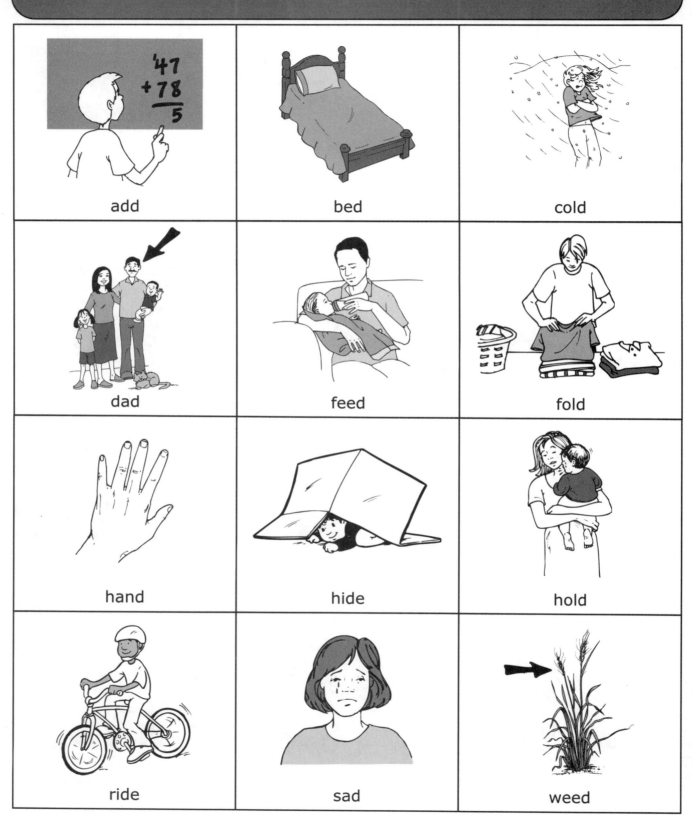

add	bed	cold
dad	feed	fold
hand	hide	hold
ride	sad	weed

Sea Creatures

Copy and cut apart the sea creatures below and on pages 164–167. Use them in April with Week Four, Activity 3 (page 112).

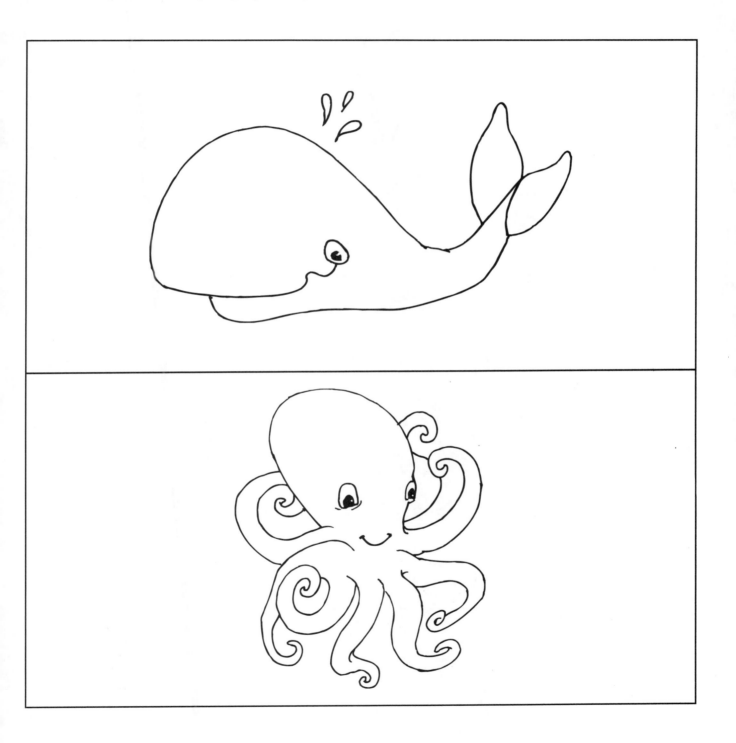

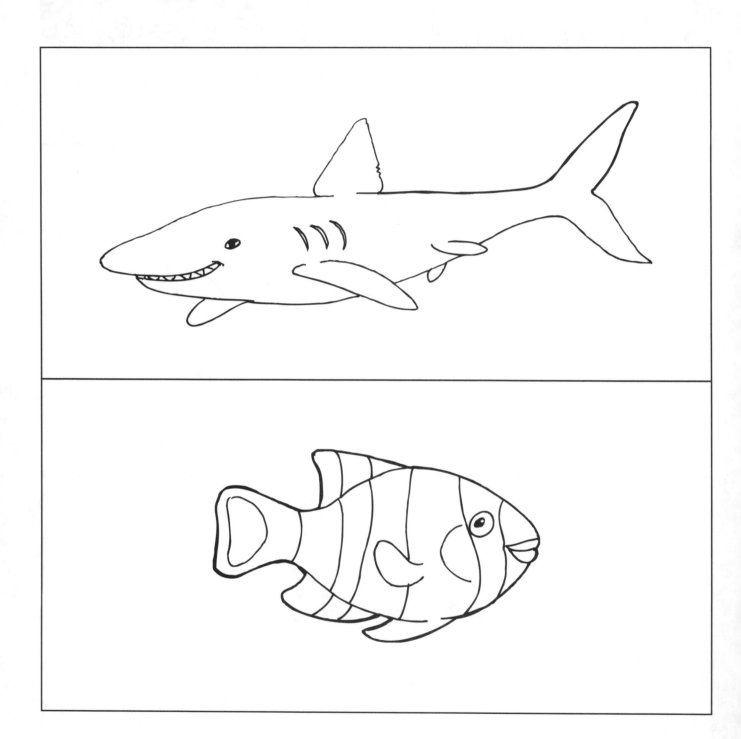

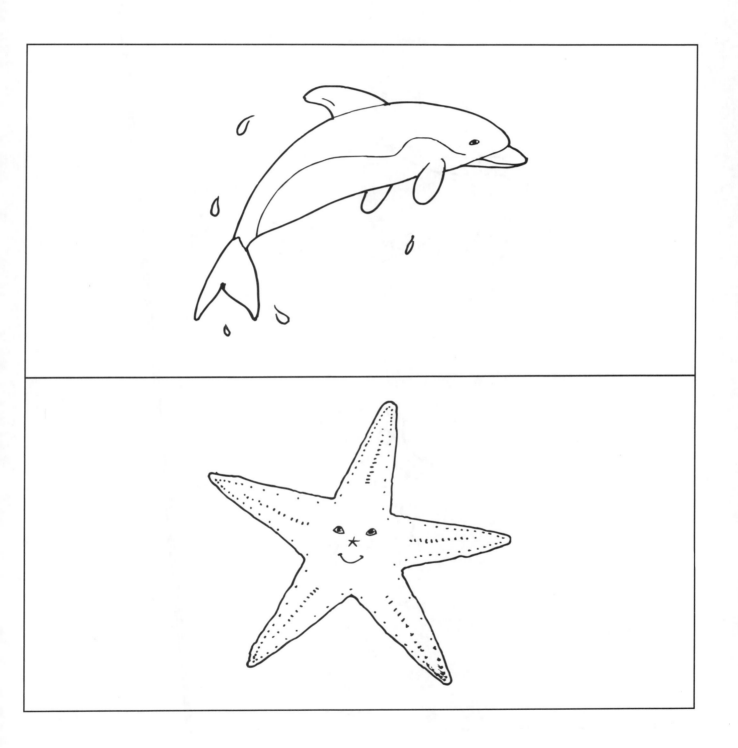

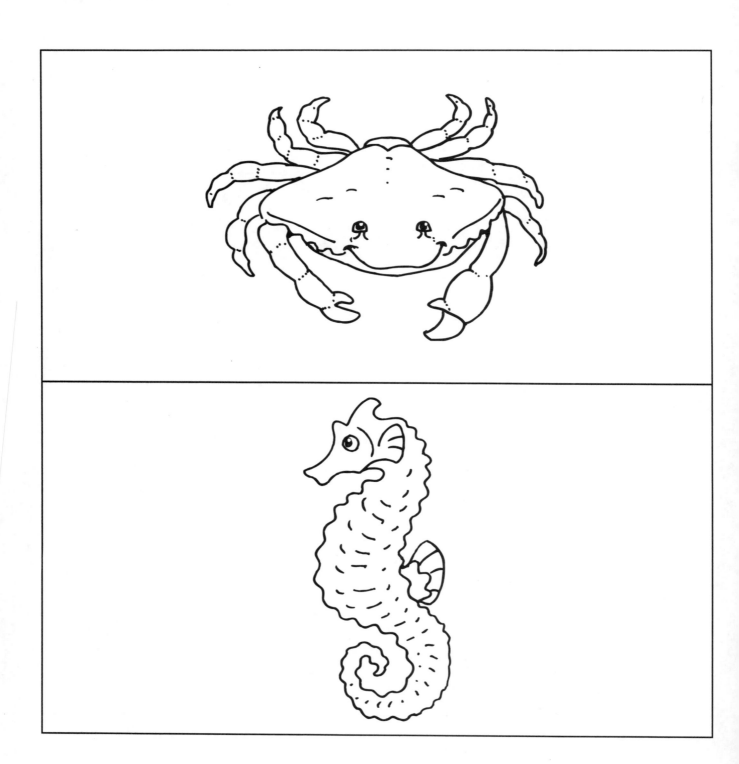

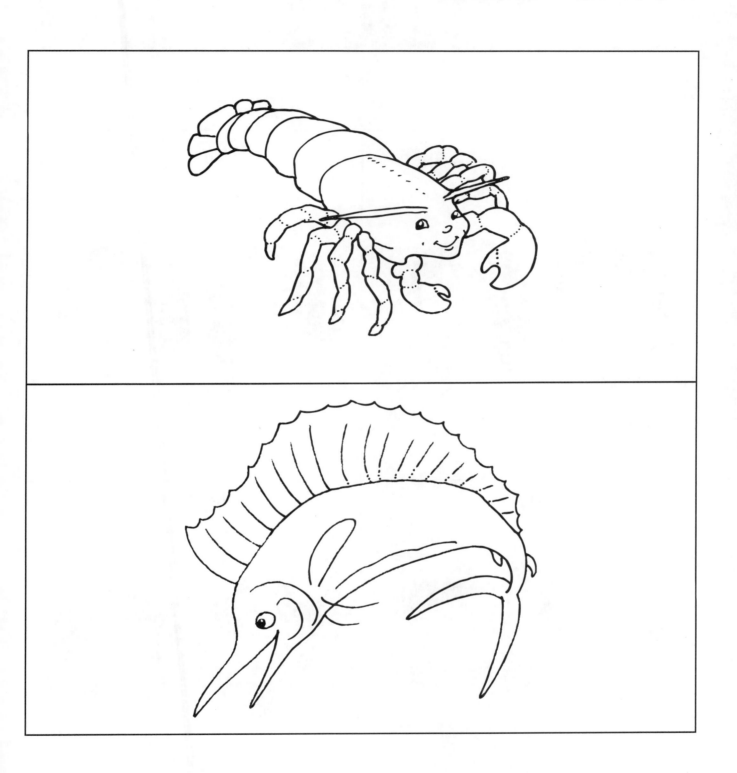

 Copyright © 2004 LinguiSystems, Inc.

Mouth Positions

Copy and cut apart the cards below and on pages 169–172. Use them in April with Week One, Activity 3 (page 102). (Note: Light bulb indicates voicing.)

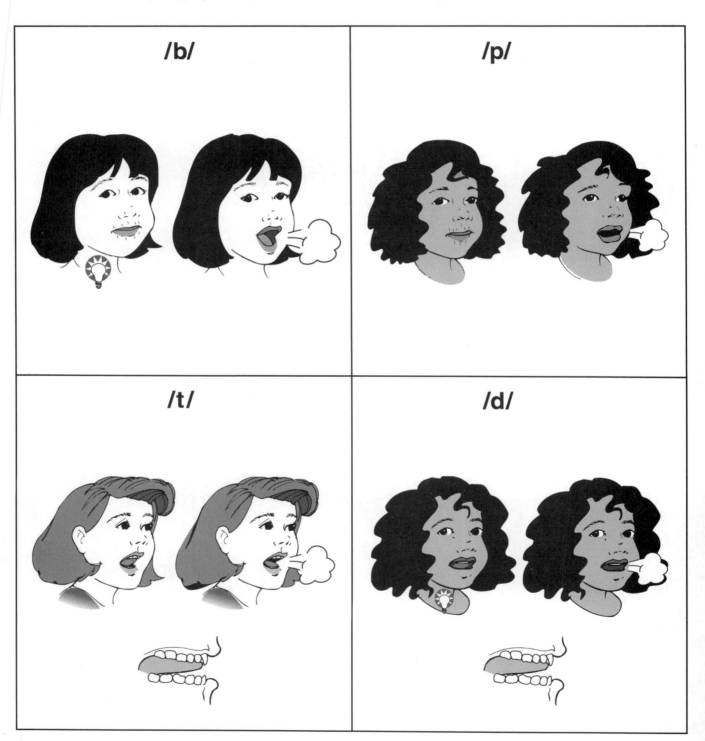

/b/

/p/

/t/

/d/

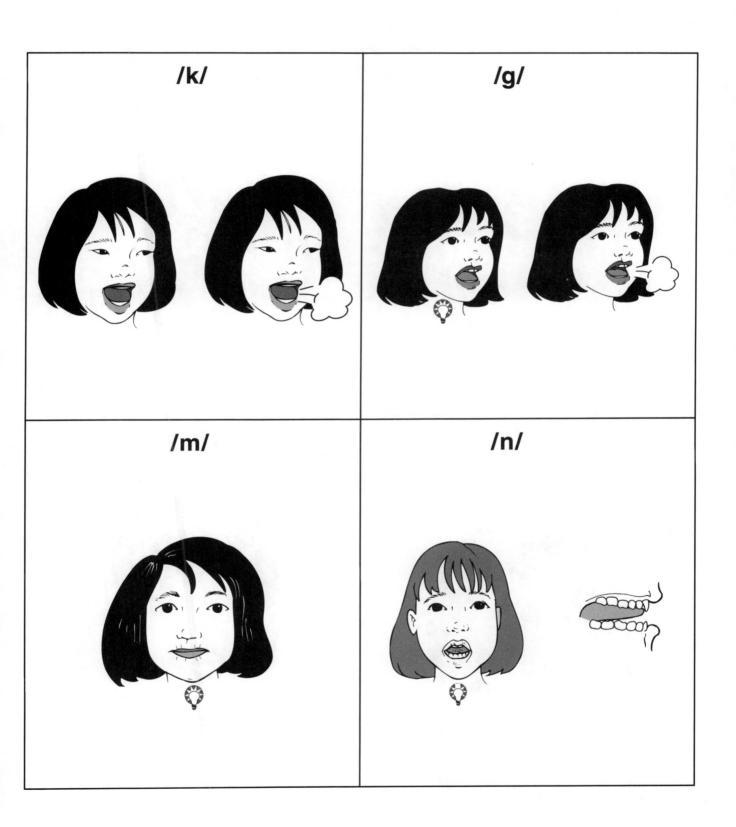

/k/

/g/

/m/

/n/

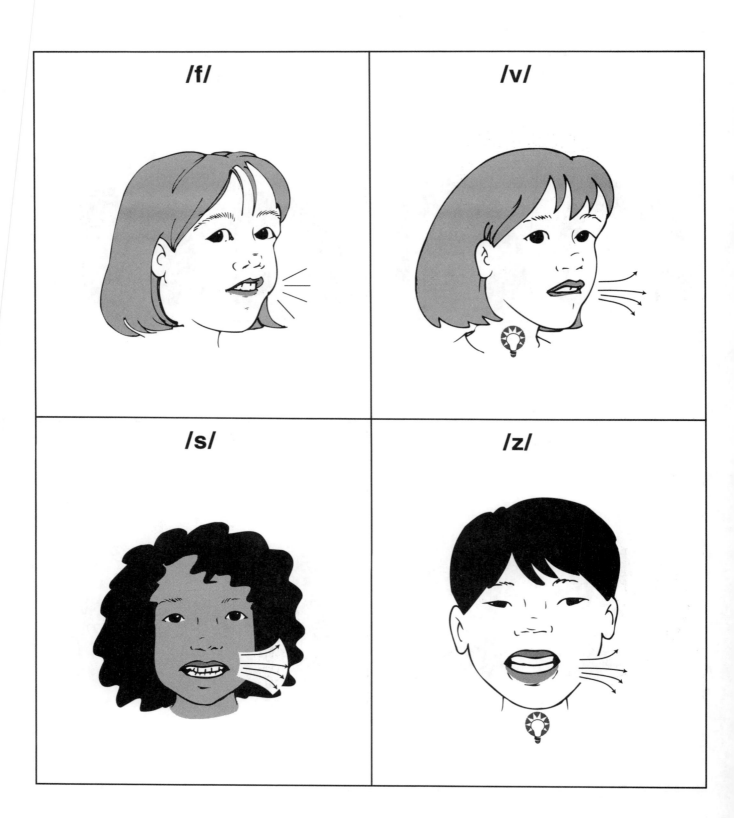

/f/

/v/

/s/

/z/

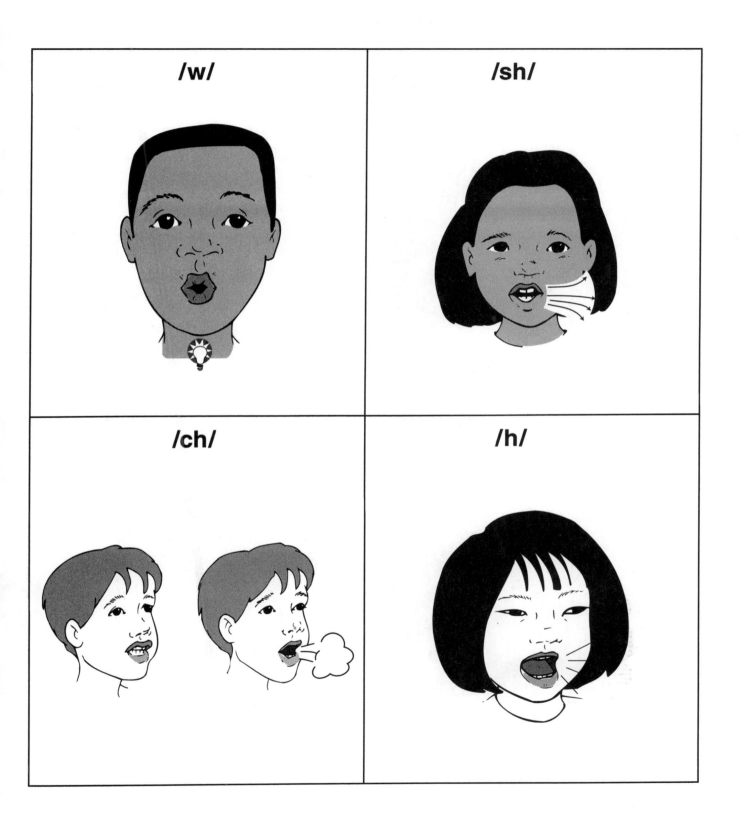

/w/

/sh/

/ch/

/h/

Copyright © 2004 LinguiSystems, Inc.

/l/ ../r/

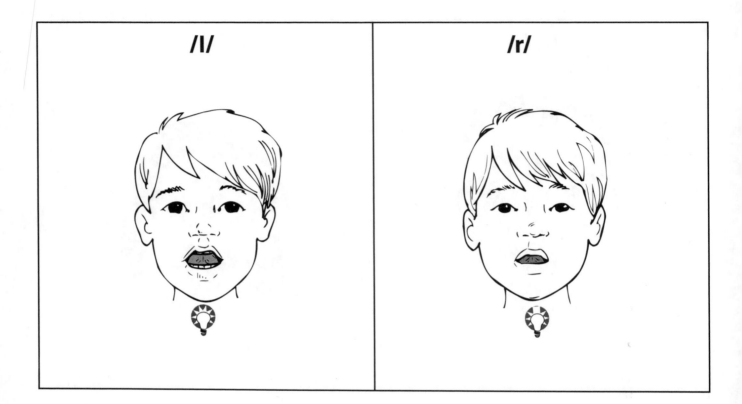

Glossary of Occupational Therapy Terms

alternating bilateral pattern	a pattern of movement when two sides of the body take turns performing equal motions in repeated sequence
bilateral pattern	a pattern of movement using both sides of the body
commando crawl	crawling with your stomach on the floor
crossing the midline	reaching from left to right or right to left, moving your arm and/or hand horizontally across an imaginary vertical line which runs from the top of your head down your nose to your belly button and then to the floor
dorsal side of hand	back of hand
finger extension	fingers straighten at all joints so hand is flat
finger flexion	fingers bend at joints toward the palm creating a fist
fingertip to palm translation (squirreling)	moving an object from fingertips to palm using the small muscles in that hand
high kneel	knees are on the floor, trunk is erect, and buttocks are off the floor to be in a high (or tall) kneel position
in-hand manipulation skills with stabilization	using the radial side of the hand while holding an object in the ulnar side of the hand
palm to fingertip translation	moving an object from palm to the fingertips with the small muscles in that hand
palmar arching	prominent arches in the palm that allow a cupping motion and grasp
palmar side of the hand	the palm side of the hand
pincer grasp	using the thumb and index finger to pick up a small object
pronation	rotate forearm so that the palm of the hand is down
prone position	lying on your stomach

 Copyright © 2004 LinguiSystems, Inc.

Glossary of Occupational Therapy Terms, *continued*

quadruped	on hands and knees in a standard crawling position
radial side of hand	thumb and pointer finger side of hand
suitcase (hook) grasp	fingers are flexed around part of an object to maintain a power hold against the object's weight or pull
supination	rotate forearm so that the palm of the hand is up facing you
supine position	lying on your back
ulnar side of hand	pinkie side of hand
wrist extension	wrist bent so the hand is raised up

 Copyright © 2004 LinguiSystems, Inc.

Picture Glossary

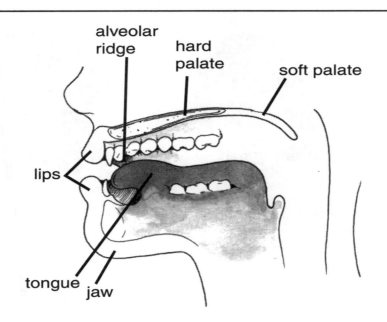

articulators for speech production

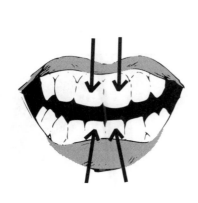

central incisors

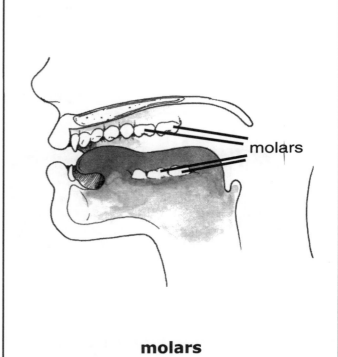

molars

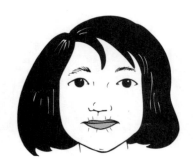 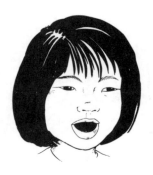

lip closure/open mouth

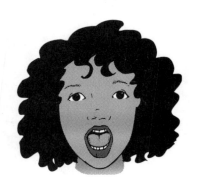

jaw drop

1st **2nd** **3rd**

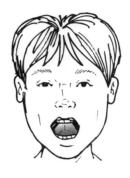 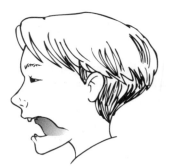 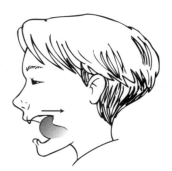

tongue elevation

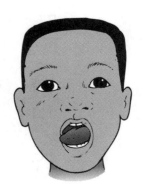 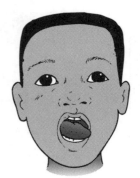

tongue lateralization

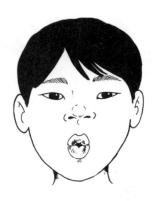

lip protrusion

Copyright © 2004 LinguiSystems, Inc.

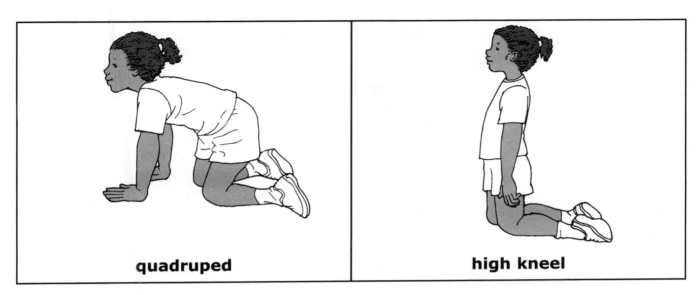

quadruped | high kneel

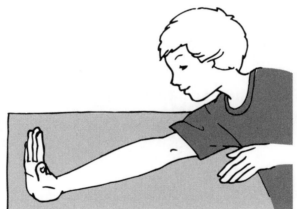

wrist extension

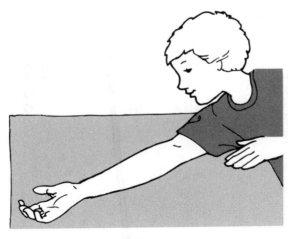

supination

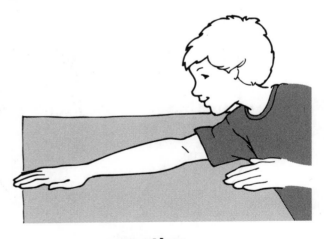

pronation

19-04-987654321

Let's Get Ready   177   Copyright © 2004 LinguiSystems, Inc.